DATE DUE

MAY 0 5 2017	

GENE THERAPY

GENE THERAPY

Evelyn B. Kelly

Health and Medical Issues Today

GREENWOOD PRESS
Westport, Connecticut • London

Library of Congress Cataloging-in-Publication Data

Kelly, Evelyn B.
    Gene therapy / Evelyn B. Kelly.
        p. cm. — (Health and medical issues today ISSN 1558–7592)
    Includes bibliographical references and index.
    ISBN 978–0–313–33760–4 (alk. paper)
        1. Gene therapy—Popular works.   2. Gene therapy—Moral and ethical aspects—
    Popular works.   I. Title.
    RB155.8.K45   2007
    616'.042—dc22   2007016143

British Library Cataloguing in Publication Data is available.

Library of Congress Catalog Card Number: 2007016143
ISBN: 978–0–313–33760–4
ISSN: 1558–7592

First published in 2007

Greenwood Press, 88 Post Road West, Westport, CT 06881
An imprint of Greenwood Publishing Group, Inc.
www.greenwood.com

Printed in the United States of America

The paper used in this book complies with the
Permanent Paper Standard issued by the National
Information Standards Organization (Z39.48–1984).

10   9   8   7   6   5   4   3   2   1

CONTENTS

Series Foreword

Every day, the public is bombarded with information on developments in medicine and health care. Whether it is on the latest techniques in treatments or research, or on concerns over public health threats, this information directly impacts the lives of people more than almost any other issue. Although there are many sources for understanding these topics—from Web sites and blogs to newspapers and magazines—students and ordinary citizens often need one resource that makes sense of the complex health and medical issues affecting their daily lives.

The *Health and Medical Issues Today* series provides just such a one-stop resource for obtaining a solid overview of the most controversial areas of health care today. Each volume addresses one topic and provides a balanced summary of what is known. These volumes provide an excellent first step for students and lay people interested in understanding how health care works in our society today.

Each volume is broken into several sections to provide readers and researchers with easy access to the information they need:

- Section I provides overview chapters on background information—including chapters on such areas as the historical, scientific, medical, social, and legal issues involved—that a citizen needs to intelligently understand the topic.
- Section II provides capsule examinations of the most heated contemporary issues and debates, and analyzes in a balanced manner the viewpoints held by various advocates in the debates.

- Section III provides a selection of reference material, including annotated primary source documents, a timeline of important events, and an annotated bibliography of useful print and electronic resources that serve as the best next step in learning about the topic at hand.

The *Health and Medical Issues Today* series strives to provide readers with all the information needed to begin making sense of some of the most important debates going on in the world today. The series will include volumes on such topics as stem-cell research, obesity, gene therapy, alternative medicine, organ transplantation, mental health, and more.

PREFACE

The popular Teenage Mutant Ninja Turtles introduced the word *mutant* into everyday language. Since publication of the first Turtles comic book in 1984, thousands of young people and adults have gasped and laughed as the powerful Turtles slashed their way through life with little concern for the reality of what a mutant is. The fact that a mutant is a gene that has changed, and the fact that the changed characteristic may be passed on to successive generations, has been totally unimportant to Turtles fans.

In fact, people throughout history—not knowing about genes and mutation—have not cared about the diseases that people are born with. Disorders and disabilities were considered simply the result of fate. Infectious diseases became the scourge of the human race when such pathogens as bubonic plague, typhoid, and typhus killed large segments of the population. However, the advent of public health programs, immunizations, and antibiotics has helped conquer most of these microbes.

Scientists in the latter half of the twentieth century were consumed with the developing science of genetics and with understanding how people inherit certain characteristics. Advances in molecular biology triggered remarkable expansion in the knowledge of human genetics and the understanding of how genes gone awry could cause diseases and disorders. The next step was logical. Some scientists in the mid-1980s began to toy with the hypothesis that if a gene causes a disease, then it should be possible to cure the disease by removing the "bad" gene and replacing it with a "good" gene. Gene therapy seemed to make sense as a logical and straightforward solution to the scourge of genetic disease. In reality, the problem is much more complex.

Misunderstanding and lack of knowledge color public perception of gene therapy. Actually, there is no one single kind of gene therapy, but many kinds of therapies dealing with different targets. As one scientist observed, "Gene therapy is
not gene therapy is not gene therapy." Although there have been setbacks and
public relations snafus, researchers are forging ahead in the belief that gene therapy is a viable and workable technique. However, the rise of these new genetic
technologies evokes concern among religious, scientific, and civic leaders that
research geneticists' immense power may spin out of control.

This book will attempt to clarify what gene therapy is and the issues related to
it. The work is organized in three sections according to the plan of Greenwood
Press's Health and Medical Issues Today series. Section One (Chapters 1 through
8) presents basic information for understanding gene therapy issues. Chapter 1
presents an overview, with background information about genetics and proteins.
Chapter 2 relates medical and scientific information necessary for understanding
gene therapy. Chapter 3 traces the history of genes as hereditary vehicles, and
details how people began to accept the idea of exchanging bad genes for good
genes. Chapter 4 traces the successes and setbacks of the 1990s and brings
research topics into the twenty-first century. Chapters 5 through 8 discuss specific
diseases and conditions that are targets for gene therapy. The chapters are arranged
according to the patterns of genetic inheritance: single-gene recessive, single-gene
dominant, X-linked conditions, and multigene conditions.

Section Two (Chapters 9 through 13) covers issues related to gene therapy,
ranging from the argumentation of ethical questions to discussion of regulatory
efforts in the United States, gene therapy developments in other countries, the
social and religious perspectives, and the future of gene therapy.

Section Three concludes the discussion with annotated primary sources, a
timeline important for the understanding of gene therapy, a glossary, sources for
further information, and an index.

This book is intended as a reference for students and other interested readers,
and attempts to describe medical and scientific concepts in common language.
Nothing in the book is intended as a substitute for medical advice. For information about personal circumstances, consult a physician or other health care professional. **Boldface** type indicates the first use of key words, which are listed in
the glossary at the end of the book.

SECTION ONE

Scientific Background of Gene Therapy

Section One, consisting of Chapters 1 through 8, presents the foundation of the science that establishes gene therapy research. This section considers the scientific background, the tools for gene therapy, the historical development of gene therapy, and the diseases and disorders targeted for research.

CHAPTER 1

Gene Therapy: A Treatment for Altered Genes

As car horns honk and taxis whiz by, the busy, crowded streets of New York City, Chicago, or Los Angeles are awhirl with bustling people—skinny and fat, light and dark, loud and quiet—scurrying like ants in all directions. Their genetics and inheritance have created the diverse ways these people look and behave. But even more startling is that each of these individuals is carrying in his or her genetic makeup about half a dozen defective, really "bad" genes. The carriers are probably blissfully unaware of this fact—unless they or their close relatives are among the millions who have a genetic disease.

Statisticians tell us that about one in ten people has or will develop a genetic disorder at some stage in life. In 1983 Victor McKusick, Professor of Medical Genetics at Johns Hopkins University, Baltimore, estimated that 2,000 to 3,000 genetic diseases can be traced to specific genes. Since that time, according to Access Excellence (1990), researchers have determined that about 2,800 of these diseases are caused by defects or mutations in just one of the patient's genes. About 2 percent of newborn infants suffer from a genetic disease. Some single-gene disorders are quite common. For example, **cystic fibrosis** is found in one in 2,500 babies born in the Western world. Other conditions, such as **ornithine transcarbamylase (OTC) deficiency,** are rare. Many other conditions, such as **Alzheimer's disease** and **Parkinson's disease,** are possibly caused by the interactions of several genes or by the gene's interaction with the environment.

Gene therapy is a medical procedure that may hold the cure for many of the diseases and disorders of humankind. Gene therapy, a rapidly growing field of medicine, is the insertion of genes into a person's cells and tissues to treat an inherited disease. It is much like a transplant. However, although transplanting a human heart or liver is complex, transferring genes involves thousands of small molecules that cannot be seen with even the most powerful of microscopes.

Gene therapy aims to supplant a defective mutant gene with a gene that works. The technology is still in its infancy but has been used with some success although many questions still surround the procedure. To understand gene therapy, it is first necessary to understand heredity.

WHAT IS A GENE?

When Robert Hooke first examined a piece of cork under a microscope, he saw structures that reminded him of prison cells. The name *cell* stuck, and even came to be applied to the 100 trillion cells that are the basic building blocks of the human organism. Over hundreds of years, scientists have struggled to find out about the cell and discovered that every cell—with a few exceptions—has a **nucleus** (the central part of the cell), a cytoplasm, and a cell membrane.

The nucleus, or central part of the cell, regulates the cells activities and has pairs of **chromosomes.** The word *chromosome* comes from two Greek root words: *chromos,* meaning "color," and *soma,* meaning "body." Under the microscope, chromosomes appear as dark-colored bodies when they are stained. Every human cell (with the exception of red blood cells, egg and sperm cells, and some cells in the bone marrow) has 23 pairs of chromosomes (46 chromosomes total), of which one pair consists of sex chromosomes. Females have two X chromosomes, whereas males have one X and one Y chromosome. The chromosomes in the other 22 pairs are called **autosomes** or **somatic,** or body chromosomes. In each pair one chromosome comes from the person's mother, the other from the person's father. Each chromosome is composed of a very long stretch of a single molecule of **deoxyribonucleic acid (DNA),** which carries the blueprint of one's heredity or genetic code. The DNA molecule looks like a twisted ladder or spiral staircase. The rungs or steps in DNA are called base pairs. Each end of a base pair is attached to a molecule of a kind of sugar, and the sugar molecules are chained together to form the sides of the ladder. There are four different kinds of base pairs, and the specific sequence of these base pairs carries information.

DNA acts like the hard drive of a computer in storing information in discrete chunks or addresses. These blocks of information are called **genes.** In a computer, the information needed to perform certain operations is provided by the software program, which is stored in a file on the hard drive and is downloaded into the random access memory (RAM), where the computer can use it to perform the operation. Relate this function to what happens in each cell. Information in the gene—a small chunk of DNA—is downloaded into **ribonucleic acid (RNA),** which, using a code, directs production of the **proteins** that make the cell work.

Transcription is the term that describes the downloading process, in which a **messenger RNA (mRNA)** molecule is formed using a single-stranded DNA template (DNA that has been temporarily unwound and the two sides of each base pair separated). The result of the process is that information contained in DNA is transferred to mRNA and this template then directs the construction of protein molecules.

This ingenious code, which appears in the form of the rungs of a ladder, is the set of sequences called nucleotides that differ by only four different bases—adenine (A), guanine (G), thymine (T), and cytosine (C) in DNA; or uracil (U) in RNA. Millions of these base pairs, or sequences, can make up a single gene. The nucleotides are made up of triplets of these bases along a strand of messenger RNA

a. The sugar-phosphate backbone is emphasized

b. Base pairs and phosphate sequences

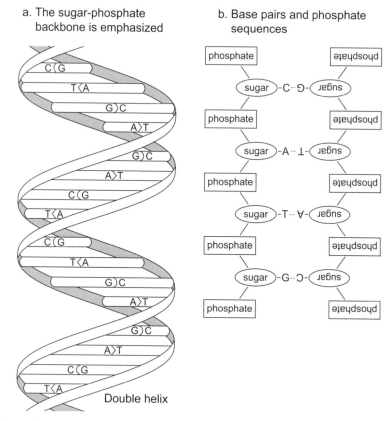

Double helix

Figure 1-1
DNA molecule.

(mRNA) that will translate into an amino acid. The three-base sequence is called a **codon.** A protein molecule is a sequence of amino acids. Thus, a gene is defined as a particular sequence of nucleotides within the DNA that specifies the sequence of **amino acids** in a particular protein. Controlling which proteins an individual cell produces will enable the gene to determine the characteristics of that cell, and ultimately determine the features of tissues, organs, and organisms.

Most genes are approximately 1,000 to 4,000 **nucleotides** in length. The entire complement of genes in a person's DNA is called the **genome.**

A PRIMER ON PROTEINS

From transcription in the mRNA, something must happen to get to the end product, which is where the process of **translation** enters in. In this process the procedure of decoding the information in the mRNA leads to directing the construction of protein molecules specified in the mRNA.

The decoding may lead to the translation of an amino acid that will create a protein. Amino acids, programmed in the genes, are the building blocks of proteins.

Proteins are long sequences or chains of amino acids. Amino acids are organic acids that contain at least one acidic carboxyl (COOH) group and one amino group (NH$_2$). More than 80 amino acids have been found in living organisms but only about 22 are considered precursors to animal proteins. Table 1-1 shows the 20 most common amino acids.

The 20 standard amino acids can be assembled in an infinite number of ways to produce a variety of proteins. The multitude of proteins in a cell perform numerous functions. The biggest single class of proteins is the **enzymes,** which are proteins that act to **catalyze,** or facilitate the building up or tearing down of, biochemical reactions. Proteins also play a part in synthesizing other proteins. One cell may contain as many as 3,000 enzymes, along with other proteins that carry messages between cells or contribute to other cell components.

The way amino acids are arranged (i.e., their sequence) determines the primary structure of the protein, which determines its function or use in the cell. However, the chain may twist, coil, and fold back on itself, making a complex

---

Meet the Human Genome

Human cell. In the human body there are about 100 trillion cells. Each cell (except red blood cells, egg and sperm cells, and some cells in the bone marrow) contains the entire human genome—the genetic information to build a human being.

Cell nucleus. Inside the cell center, about 6 feet of deoxyribonucleic acid (DNA) are packaged into 23 pairs of chromosomes, with one chromosome in each pair coming from each parent.

Chromosome. Each of the 46 human chromosomes contains the DNA for thousands of individual genes, the units of heredity.

Gene. Each gene is a segment of double-stranded DNA that holds the "recipe" for making a specific molecule, usually a protein. These recipes are spelled out in varying sequences of the four chemical bases in DNA: adenine (A), thymine (T), guanine (G), and cytosine (C). A DNA molecule looks like two ladders, each with a side taken off and then twisted around one another. The rungs of the ladder meet, forming a spiral staircase-like structure known as base pairs. The bases form interlocking pairs that fit together in one way: A pairs with T, G pairs with C. Millions of these base pairs or sequences can make up a single gene. These genes ultimately direct an organism's growth and characteristics through the production of the chemical proteins.

Protein. Proteins are made up of amino acids and are the essential components of all organs and chemical activities. Their functions depend on their shape and are determined by the 30,000 genes in the cell nucleus.

and intricate molecule. This shape is dependent on the amino acid composition; any change in just a single amino acid can have a profound effect on the protein and its function.

It is amazing that from only four letters of the four bases of a DNA molecule, 20 or more amino acids and thousands of proteins can be assembled. The ingenious three-letter system, or code, is based on three nucleotides. Each triplet, or codon, specifies one amino acid. For example, AAA—that is adenine, adenine, adenine—is a sequence that will code for the amino acid lysine, and CCC—cytosine, cytosine, cytosine—codes for proline. The number of combinations is 4^3 (or four cubed, or 64). There are at least three times as many codons as are necessary to encode 20 amino acids. In fact, many amino acids are encoded by multiple codons, and one codon may signal the starting point for protein translation and three stop codons may signal the end of translation.

In addition, a gene is more than just the amino acid sequences of a protein. Relate the gene to a recipe for baking chocolate chip cookies. The sequences are the list of ingredients, but information on what and how to mix, how to add the ingredients, and how long to bake the cookies is included. The gene does the same things. There are sections of the genes, such as **promoters** and **introns,** which contain all the information as to when to make the protein, how much to make, and when to stop. For example, the DNA sequence that codes for human insulin is more than 4,000 bases long; yet insulin is a small protein of only about

Table 1-1   The 20 Most Common Amino Acids

Name	Shorthand
Glycine	Gly
Alanine	Ala
Valine	Val
Leucine	Leu
Isoleucine	Iso
Serine	Ser
Theronine	Thr
Cysteine	Cys
Methionine	Met
Aspartic acid	Asp
Asparagine	Asn
Glutamic acid	Glu
Glutamine	Glu
Lysine	Lys
Arginine	Arg
Histidine	His
Phenyalanine	Phe
Tyrosine	Tyr
Tryptophan	Trp
Proline	Pro

Table created by Evelyn Kelly.

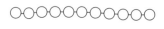

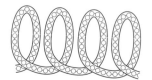

Primary structure - Amino
acids in polypeptide chain

Secondary structure - loops,
coils, helices, barrels or sheets
when amino acids attract

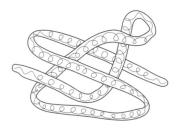

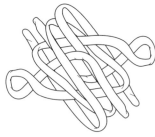

Tertiary structure - Folds occur
in the secondary structure

Quaterary structure - several
folds

Figure 1-2
Picture of a protein.

100 amino acids. Complex instructions in the recipe include how to make this molecule. Projects are now underway to completely analyze and understand the human **proteome,** the complete set of proteins that make up the body. This task is even more challenging than deciphering the human genome.

In summary, DNA is not directly involved in protein synthesis. If the DNA is unzipped or the double chain comes apart, the information is transcribed into messenger RNA (mRNA). Rather than directions making a complementary strand of DNA, a template is used to make a matching strand of RNA, which is identical except it contains a ribose sugar, and thymine is replaced by uracil. The RNA with the copy of the genetic code leaves the nucleus (where the process has been going on) and enters the cytoplasm of the cells. Here it binds to a protein part of the cell called the ribosome.

The mRNA–ribosome partnership then carries out the DNA's instructions to make or translate the synthesis of the protein. Codons along the mRNA synthesized from the DNA template control the sequence of the insertions of amino acids into the protein chain during the process of translation. Note that it is the RNA messenger (mRNA) that encodes and determines that the correct sequence of amino acids is encoded in the process called transcription.

DISEASES OF GENETIC ORIGIN

Many things can go wrong in the translation process. Think of the process of a group of workers on an assembly line making peanut butter sandwiches. Each person has a job to do: unwrapping the loaf of bread, spreading the peanut butter, spreading the jelly, putting the top and bottom slices of bread together. The process moves rapidly like clockwork. But suppose the worker spreading the jelly drops his knife and has to go under the table to retrieve it. The assembly line people keep doing their jobs, but no jelly is spread on the next sandwich. Now it is only a peanut butter sandwich. This simple illustration shows how just one small slip can change the outcome of a product. Likewise, even small changes in the primary structure of a protein may have a large effect on the protein's properties.

Single-gene Trait or Mendelian Traits

The diseases most likely to be treated with gene therapy are probably those caused by mutations in a single gene. Such diseases are called single-gene defects and contrast with diseases that are caused by multiple genes and environmental factors. A single misplaced amino acid can alter a protein's function. Take the example of the genetic disease **sickle cell anemia.** A single molecule of valine has replaced the glutamic acid molecule in one of the chains of the **hemoglobin** molecule, the protein that carries oxygen in the red blood cells. This tiny error causes a misshaped molecule and deformity in the carrying capacity of the red blood cells.

The single-gene trait obeys relatively simple laws of inheritance—the laws determined by the monk Gregor Mendel, who lived in the nineteenth century and

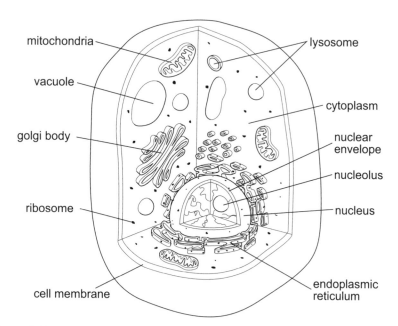

Figure 1-3
The cell and its parts.

who described patterns of inheritance in plants. These same genetic inheritance patterns apply to genetic diseases such as cystic fibrosis and **Huntington's disease.**

The single-gene trait can be classified according to a number of disorders and traits:

- *Recessive disorders.* Conditions occur when one receives a defective gene from both parents. Most of these diseases occur when dysfunctional gene pairs produce protein abnormalities that cause chemical imbalances. In general, if the harmful gene is recessive, one normal gene masks the defective gene to avoid all symptoms of disease. Only if one inherits the same recessive genes from both parents will the disease develop. These diseases are probably the best understood because they can be traced to the defects in a specific enzyme.
- *Dominant disorders.* When an offspring receives a defective gene from just one parent, the condition may appear. The molecular effect in dominant conditions is less well established than in recessive ones.
- *X-linked disorders.* These disorders are carried on the X chromosome and usually appear in males because no set of second genes on a second X chromosomes masks the defective copy. The pattern of inheritance is distinctive: a son inherits the traits only from his mother because the X chromosome is from the mother and the Y that made the son a male is from the father. Daughters can get the defective gene from either parent but usually do not have the disease unless they get the abnormal gene from both parents. Apparently, few traits and no known diseases are carried on the Y chromosome.
- *Multigene traits.* The interaction of several genes can cause certain traits. Genes specify eye and hair color but do not follow simple Mendelian patterns. Such disorders are termed polygenic or multigene.
- *Environmentally modified traits.* The combination of genetic predisposition and interaction with the environment determines the vast majority of characteristics. For example, height is influenced by nutrition and other factors. Many diseases derive from the interaction of genes with the environment. For example, heart disease, cancer, and many drug reactions appear to involve multiple genes as well as environmental influences.

Genes are carried on chromosomes and are the basic physical and functional units of heredity. They contain the chemical information that makes cells work and instruct cellular material to produce proteins vital to the cell's function. The genetic code is a set of very specific sequences of bases that encode instructions on how to make proteins. A protein is the product of the expression of a gene. One slight change or mutation may garble the protein-making instructions, resulting in a genetic disease. Therefore, identifying, isolating, and studying genes and their functions is a powerful approach to a better understanding of diseases. Chapters 5 through 8 discuss some specific conditions that occur when genes are mutated.

What Is Gene Therapy?

Gene therapy is a set of approaches designed to correct the defective genes responsible for disease development. The technique is based on the transfer of a "normal" gene into an individual's cells and tissues to treat an "abnormal" hereditary disease-causing gene. Several questions should be considered before undertaking gene therapy:

- Does the condition result from changes in one or more genes?
- Do researchers know where the gene is located?
- Can copies of the gene be made in the laboratory?
- What is known about the disorder? What tissues does it affect? Is there a protein known to be related to the disorder?
- Will adding a normal copy of the gene fix the problem?
- Do scientists have the ability to effectively deliver functioning genes into cells where the gene defect exists?

Gene therapy is actually a sophisticated extension of conventional medical therapy. Rather than treat a patient's disease with drugs or surgery, the patient receives DNA. Several approaches may be used for correcting the defect:

- *Gene insertion.* A normal gene may be inserted into a nonspecific location within the genome to replace a nonfunctional gene. This approach is the most common.
- *Gene modification.* An abnormal gene may be swapped for a normal gene using recombination.
- *Gene surgery.* The abnormal gene may be repaired through reverse mutation or by changing the defect to return the gene to normal function.
- *Gene regulation.* The degree to which a gene is turned on or off may be altered. For example, certain genes may regulate the process of the production of proteins. Targets to change regulation of these genes are a possibility.

Types of Gene Therapy

Gene therapy seeks to supplant genes that are not doing their job. It is theoretically possible at two levels to transfer somatic cells and germ-line cells such as sperm, ova, and their **stem cell** precursors:

- *Somatic gene therapy.* This type introduces therapeutic genes at the tissue or cellular level to treat a specific individual. Only the person receiving the treatment is affected. There are two categories of somatic gene therapy:

    1. **Ex vivo (or in vitro) therapy,** in which cells are modified outside the body for later transplantation back into the body.
    2. **In vivo therapy,** in which genes are changed in cells still in the body.

- *Germ-line gene therapy.* In this form of therapy, genes are inserted into the reproductive cells or possibly into embryos to treat diseases that could be passed on to successive generations. This is the more controversial of the two forms. Some people fear that germ-line therapy could be used to control human development in ways not connected with disease (e.g., to control development on the basis of an individual's intelligence or appearance).

THE HUMAN GENOME PROJECT

Great strides have been made in applications of gene therapy in a short period of time, yet lack of scientific data limits its useful potential. The control of the functions of the human body is not simple. For example, the vast majority of genetic material does not store information for the creation of proteins but is involved in the control and regulation of gene expression. Some of these pathways are very complex and difficult to interpret. To fully understand the pathways, scientists must discover the biological role of individual genes and learn where the base pairs that make them are located in the DNA. In April 2003 the finished sequence was announced, with 99 percent of the human genome's gene-containing regions mapped to an accuracy of 99.9 percent. The genes identified in the Human Genome project include a gene that predisposes people to obesity; one associated with programmed cell death (i.e., apoptosis); a gene that guides HIV viral reproduction; and the genes of inherited disorders like Huntington's disease, Lou Gehrig's disease, and some colon and breast cancers. Chapter 3 relates the history of the development of the genome project. Chapters 5 through 8 present some specific diseases and current trials.

Although gene therapy is simple in concept, obstacles and challenges have proven to be quite demanding. Chapter 2 addresses the medical and scientific challenges of gene therapy.

CHAPTER 2

Medical and Scientific Issues in Gene Therapy

Kary Mullis, a biochemist working for the California biotechnology firm Cetus, cruised along Highway 128 from San Francisco to Mendicino. Somehow, he found he could think about solving problems while driving his Honda Civic. That day in 1970 was like any other travel day for Kary Mullis, until he was struck by the idea of how to make many copies of a gene fragment. It was so simple; he wondered why he hadn't seen it before. He envisioned a chain reaction in which copies are made in a machine. For this idea, known as polymerase chain reaction (PCR), he was awarded the Nobel Prize in Chemistry in 1993. PCR is one of the tools at the foundation of gene therapy.

Imagine a 5-year-old boy who is determined to build a house. He is given a very expensive toolbox full of the latest technological materials. He desires to build the most beautiful house according to the architect's plans. The will is there, but the know-how and experience are not. The present state of gene therapy can be likened to a toolbox in the hands of a novice carpenter. The instruments, devices, and tools are there. Scientists have just not been able to master them yet to do everything that may be possible.

The toolbox of gene therapy involves three main elements:

- Isolating the gene of interest
- Putting the gene into the cells where it will be used
- Ensuring that the inserted gene functions in the new cells in a way that does not harm the patient.

ISOLATING AND COPYING THE GENE

Genetic information gets into new cells by duplication or mitosis. In mitosis the cell divides copying its DNA and giving a copy to each of the new offspring cells. The Human Genome Project identified the organization of bases in DNA as adenine–thymine–cytosine–guanine (ATCG). It also determined there are about 30,000 genes—a surprise because scientists had previously assumed there were more then 100,000 genes. If the dividing cell carries the DNA for a mutated, disease-producing gene, that gene will be passed on in the genome. Identifying the abnormal gene is essential.

Polymerase Chain Reaction

To be able to accomplish gene therapy copies of the normal gene are made. The process of making multiple copies of a single gene in the laboratory is called **cloning.** The process of polymerase chain reaction (PCR) enables repetitive DNA replication over a limited region in the DNA where the known gene is located.

The PCR machine looks like a simple, unimpressive box with a lot of buttons and knobs. For PCR to occur, four things must be present: a template, primer, the four nucleotides (adenine, thymine, cytosine, and guanine), and DNA polymerase. **Primers** are engineered pieces of DNA of 18 to 24 bases that are made to lie between another stretch of DNA that is destined to be copied. When a class of enzymes called restriction enzymes cuts open a particular nucleotide sequence, the primer binds to the exposed single-stranded region of DNA. DNA polymerase is present in normal cell division to duplicate the entire DNA and pass a copy to each daughter cell. The process in nature is called replication.

Steps in PCR are as follows

1. The targeted double-stranded DNA is heated to 194°F, and the strands are separated from each other and made ready to be used as a template.
2. At the lowered temperature of 120°F, primers attach or anneal to their complementary sequence on each template.
3. The nucleotides then extend the primer.
4. At the end of each cycle, the number of DNA molecules doubles.

Although the cycles were at one time manually controlled, theromocyclers are now designed to automatically change temperatures. The heat cycle comes from an unusual source. The bacterium *Thermus aquaticus,* found in the hot springs of Yellowstone National Park, provided a high-temperature-resistant DNA polymerase. PCR is valuable to researchers because it enables them to multiply unique DNA sequences in a short period of time. This first step of multiplying the gene is exceedingly important in gene therapy.

INSERTION INTO HUMAN CELLS

To transport the entire gene or a recombinant DNA to the cell's nucleus requires molecular "delivery trucks" called **vectors.** One usually thinks of a vector such as an insect that carries some infectious disease from a host to an individual. By analogy, a genetically disabled virus used in gene therapy is referred to as a vector because it carries genes to the cell. All vectors have one thing in common: the delivery and insertion of therapeutic material into cells. Here the similarities end.

Viruses as Vectors

Viruses—those sneaky little microbes that have caused such havoc by causing smallpox, typhus, and the great scourges of history—are really simple little organisms. Those with only a few genes are usually single-stranded ribonucleic acid (RNA), whereas those with more genes have double-stranded DNA. Viruses may appear as single-stranded RNA, double-stranded DNA, double-stranded RNA, single-stranded DNA, or circular. In double-stranded genomes, one of the strands provides protection and stability with the other codes for working genes.

All viruses are cellular parasites that cannot replicate their genome without other cells. An animal cell has a nucleus, cytoplasm, and cell membrane; plants have the same structure except each cell is surrounded by a cell wall. To secure entry into the cell, sugar and some hormone molecules have receptors that link to the cell in a process called **endocytosis,** or taking into the cell. One of the great talents of the virus is to form a **capsid,** a small vesicle that connects with these receptors and is drawn into the cell. When it gets inside it releases an enzyme that spews the virus chromosome into the cytoplasm. Some viruses vary this process. For example, HIV fuses with the cell membrane and then releases the capsid directly into the cytoplasm.

Because of their ability to sneak into cells, viruses appear to be efficient delivery vehicles for replacing mutant genes. But first three major obstacles stand in the way:

1. Scientists must find a way to block the ability of the virus to replicate its own genome.
2. They must stop the production of viral messenger RNA that codes for the proteins that help the virus escape into the cell.
3. They must insert the therapeutic gene in such a way that the formation of the capsid will be normal, allowing the virus to get into the cell.

All the action takes place in a test tube (i.e., ex vivo). The viral genes for infection are taken out and then the therapeutic gene is inserted into the viral chromosome. The hybrid is then mixed with purified viral capsid proteins. If the procedure is performed properly, the virus carrying its payload gene will be able to get into the cell but will not harm it.

Following are the most common vectors currently under investigation:

- *Retroviruses.* The genetic material in retroviruses is in the form of RNA molecules, while the genetic material of the hosts is in the form of DNA. When a retrovirus infects a host cell, it introduces its RNA together with some enzymes into the cell. The RNA molecule must produce a DNA copy from its RNA molecule before it can be considered part of the genetic material of the host cell. Retroviruses are a class of virus that can create double-stranded DNA copies of their RNA genomes. Because the genetic material is RNA rather than DNA, retroviruses produce an enzyme known as **reverse transcriptase.** Because they make this enzyme, they can transform their RNA into DNA, which can be permanently integrated into the DNA of the host cells. Scientists were the first to use these vectors, which are easily cloned and work best in actively dividing cells. Critical retroviral genes are removed so that the virus cannot reproduce after it delivers its genetic cargo. However, because cells in the body do not divide often, retroviruses are used primarily ex vivo (i.e., outside the body). The process works in the following way:

1. Cells are first removed from the patient's body so that the virus or the vector carrying the gene can be inserted into them.
2. The cells are placed in a nutrient culture where they grow and replicate.
3. When there are a sufficient number of cells, they are injected into the bloodstream. As long as these cells survive, they will provide the desired therapy. These viruses, including HIV, incorporate their passenger genes into nondividing cells such as those of the brain or liver (although some scientists are skeptical about using a deadly virus for therapeutic purposes). The ex vivo requirement and the necessity to divide the cells are the disadvantages of working with retroviruses. The retrovirus known as mouse (or *murine,* pertaining to mice or rats) leukemia virus (MuLV) has been used in many gene therapy trials.

- *Adenoviruses.* This class of virus has double-stranded DNA genomes that cause respiratory, intestinal, and eye infections in humans. They efficiently enter most cells and can infect stationary cells. Advantages of working with this class of virus include high levels of replication and expression, ease of handling, and their capacity to infect many types of human cells, including nondividing ones. A disadvantage of working with adenoviruses is that the immune system responds, and expels the foreign material from the body. Researchers are trying to move large portions of unessential DNA, hoping the body will not reject the virus and its payload. The virus that causes the common cold is an adenovirus. Adenovirus type 2 (AD-2) has been used in trials targeting **T lymphocytes** (the cells of the immune system) and a number of tumor cells. A form of AD-2 has been therapeutically injected directly into the liver for treatment. The problem here is tricky. Too little will cause insufficient gene expression; too much can infect other cells. Also, the expression of the therapeutic gene tends to decline after a week or so.
- *Adeno-associated viruses (AAVs).* These viruses are small, single-stranded DNA viruses that can insert their genetic material at a specific site on chromosome 19. They cause no known diseases in humans and have long-term expression. They have the ability to target nondividing cells located in muscle and in the brain, liver, and lungs, and can insert their genome into the genome of the recipient. They also appear to evade the assault of the immune system. Because of their staying power, they hold promise for the treatment of such chronic diseases as hemophilia. A 2006 study by scientists at the University of Florida evaluated a method of delivering three subtypes of adeno-associated virus, which are not known to trigger an immune response reaction. They tested the ability of AAV-1, AAV-8, and AAV-9 to insert genes

into skeletal and heart muscle. Tests revealed that AAV-9 was taken into the heart in amounts 200 times the level at which AAV was taken in.

- *Lentiviruses.* Lentiviruses (LVs) are derived from a special group of viruses, of which HIV is a member. HIV has adapted itself to enter human cells in an effective manner. For this reason HIV has been difficult to eradicate, but for the same reason, the virus may develop into be a very efficient vector. Researchers must engineer a way to make virus vectors less dangerous. For example, removing just six genes from HIV makes it less virulent. LVs have been evaluated in clinical human trials. A Phase I trial for the treatment of patients with HIV/AIDS was successfully completed at the University of Pennsylvania, which showed excellent safety profiles.

LVs have vast potential as drug discovery tools, including their possible use in target validation and in generation of engineered cell lines and transgenic animals. However, here perception becomes part of the problem. Who wants a debilitated HIV virus injected into his or her body?

- *Herpesviruses.* Herpesviruses can deliver chunks of DNA up to ten times the size of other vectors. They can be produced in high concentration and are neurotropic (i.e., are drawn to the nervous system). Projected uses are in the treatment of such neurological disorders as brain tumors.
- *Poxviruses.* These viruses, which reproduce in large numbers, can insert sizable chunks of DNA with high expression. However, they are targets of the immune system.

Nonviral Methods

At meetings of such medical associations as the American Society for Gene Therapy, debate often centers on which vectors will prevail. The newer field of nonviral vectors suggests several novel approaches to gene therapy:

- *Naked DNA.* The simplest of all methods involves use of naked DNA, which is easy to prepare in large quantities and has high safety levels in tests thus far. This vector is injected into the muscle. The amount of naked DNA that can be injected is unlimited because it can deliver larger chunks of DNA and cause relatively less severe immune reactions. However, the usefulness of naked DNA appears to be limited by a low rate of gene transfer and lower gene efficiency compared to viruses. Because naked DNA does not integrate into the cells, its projected use may be for mechanical and topical applications and for accessible areas such as skin, vascular, pulmonary, and endothelial cells. Use by in vivo vaccination appears to be promising. A newer method of delivery has been the **gene gun,** which shoots DNA-coated gold particles into cells using high-pressure gas.
- *Facilitated DNA or* **liposomes.** Direct administration of DNA or DNA complexes such as liposomes in vivo is in its infancy. Here an artificial lipid sphere with an aqueous core is created that can carry therapeutic DNA. The

vector could carry genes of unlimited size, but its low efficiency compared with viruses and the absence of a mechanism to maintain the therapeutic effect are drawbacks. Recently, newer molecules—lipoplexes and polyplexes—have been created that can protect DNA from degrading during the insertion process. The most common use of lipoplexes has been in gene transfer into cancer cells.

- *Human artificial chromosomes.* The idea of building a chromosome from the ground up—using a set of telomeres, a centrosome, and therapeutic material—could mimic one advantage of the herpes-based vector without the toxicity. This chromosome would be capable of carrying substantial amounts of genetic code and the immune system would not attach to it. It could carry a large insertion of multiple genes, which of course would be the downfall of this method—its delivery of such a large molecule to the nucleus of a target cell.
- *Infectious mammalian chromosomes.* This technique represents a synthesis of viral and nonviral approaches. Researchers produced a component of the Epstein-Barr virus (EBV) in the form of a large circular molecule that shows stable expression for longer than a year. EBV is a very large virus belonging to the herpes family. In early transgenic studies, the efficiency of this method was 25 percent higher than strictly nonviral vectors.
- *Starburst dendrites and new polymers.* These polymers are shaped like a star. Partially fractured versions have the ability to release DNA from the endosomes, a quality lacking in some nonviral approaches.
- *Endothelial cells.* Modifying endothelial cells into vectors could provide a specific delivery system. Harvested from subcutaneous fat or even the bloodstream, endothelial cells are readily available.

Hybrid Methods

Because every method may have shortcomings, some hybrid methods combine two or more techniques. **Virsomes** combine liposomes with an inactivated HIV or influenza virus. This method has been more effective in gene transfer in respiratory epithelial cells than methods based on viral and epithelial cells alone. Many scientists think that the debate over viruses and nonviruses will merge and that the best vector will probably be a hybrid. Of the systems studied to date, retroviruses appear to be the best suited for gene therapy, although new information about vectors and new approaches emerge almost weekly.

Other Approaches

What happens if adding a "good" copy of a gene does not solve the problem of mutation or defect? If the mutated gene encodes a protein that prevents a normal protein from doing its job, then just adding a normal gene will not help. Mutated genes that function in this way are called dominant negative. Repairing the gene or getting rid of it completely may be one solution. The RNA therapeutics company Intronn Inc. has developed a technique for repairing mutations that it calls SMaRT™, or spliceosome-mediated RNA *trans*-splicing. Remember from Chapter 1 that messenger RNA makes transcripts copied from mutated genes. Instead of trying to replace the entire gene, the SMaRT approach targets and repairs just the section of the mRNA transcript that is mutated. A human gene contains regions called **exons** that encode the protein, and regions called **introns** that do not encode the protein. When the gene is copied into mRNA, the RNA machinery uses spliceosomes to cut out the noncoding parts and splice together the coding parts. The SMaRT technology involves delivering an RNA start that pairs with the intron next to the mutated segment of mRNA. This prevents spliceosomes from including the mutated segment in the final RNA product. At the same time, a correct version of the segment replaces the mutated section in the final mRNA product, and the repaired mRNA produces a normal, properly functioning protein.

TECHNIQUES TO PREVENT PRODUCTION OF MUTATED PROTEINS

Several techniques—therapies involving triple-helix-forming oligonucleotides, antisense, and ribozymes—are used to stop the production of a mutated gene and keep the mutated cell from being copied.

- Triple-helix-forming **oligonucleotide** gene therapy targets the DNA sequence of a mutated gene to prevent its transcription. Transcription is the process by which a complementary mRNA molecule is formed from a single-stranded DNA template. The information in the DNA is transferred to the mRNA, which is then used as a template to direct the construction of a protein. Triple-helix-forming oligonucleotide therapy uses a short, single-stranded piece of DNA that binds right into the groove between the double strands of the mutated gene's DNA. The triple-helix that is produced prevents the segment of DNA from being transcribed into mRNA.

- **Antisense gene therapy** turns off a mutated gene in a cell by targeting the mRNA transcripts copied from the gene. Genes are made of two paired strands of DNA. During transcription, the sequence of one strand is copied into a single strand of mRNA, which is called the *sense strand* in that it has the code to be read for making the protein. The opposite is called the *antisense strand*. Procedures to perform this therapy involve delivery of an RNA strand containing the antisense code of a mutated gene and binding the antisense RNA strands to the mutated sense mRNA strands, preventing the mRNA from being translated into a mutated protein.

- **Ribozyme** therapy turns off a mutated gene by targeting transcripts copied from the gene, thus preventing the production of the mutated protein. Ribozymes are RNA molecules that act like enzymes, serving as scissors to cut RNA. Ribozyme therapy involves delivering the RNA strands that have been engineered to function as ribozymes, where they bind to mRNA encoded by the mutated gene. There the ribozyme cuts off the target RNA and prevents it from being translated into a protein.

How are these highly controversial and experimental procedures tested? Human testing is very rigidly controlled, but animal models of disease are widely used to test new therapies, and trials are proceeding cautiously, viral vectors still being the most common. The types of vectors used in 2006 in gene therapy trials are presented in Table 2-1.

ENSURING THAT THE PATIENT WILL NOT BE HARMED

Here comes the tricky part of gene therapy—actually getting the gene into the patient while ensuring that he or she is done no harm. The decision to follow a given gene therapy protocol depends on the satisfaction of several requirements. Safeguards are imposed to ensure the safety, efficacy, and reliability of gene therapy procedures; that alternative treatments have been explored; that the severity of symptoms and prognosis have been evaluated; and that informed consent has been freely given. See the sidebar, Phases Leading to Food and Drug Administration Approval.

Table 2-1 Vectors in Gene Therapy Trials

Vector	Number of Trials Using Vector
Adenovirus	305
Retrovirus	228
Naked or plasmid DNA	206
Lipofection (liposomes)	99
Poxvirus	82
Vaccinia virus	78
Adeno-associated virus	40
Herpes simplex virus	40
RNA transfer	15
Lentivirus	6
Flavivirus	5
Gene gun	5
Adenovirus + retrovirus	3
Measles virus	3
Saccaromyces cerevisiae	2
Salmonella typhimurium	2
Listeria monocutogenes	1
Naked or plasmid DNA + adenovirus	1
Newcastle disease virus	1
Poliovirus	1
Semliki Forest virus	1
Simian virus 40	1
Recombinant pox virus	1
Unknown	37
Total	1192

Adapted by Evelyn B. Kelly from materials in *The Journal of Gene Medicine,* updated July 2006.

Phases Leading to Food and Drug Administration Approval

Research phase	Goals of the Trials
Preclinical research	This is the basic research phase, during which the idea for treatment is tested in many trials, generally using such small animals as mice. With the animal model of the disease or disorder developed, the experiments are replicated many times. After mice, experiments may extend to such larger animals as dogs, pigs, or monkeys.[1]
Phase I	After preclinical research, applications are made to the FDA, the National Institutes of Health (NIH), and the Recombinant DNA Advisory Committee (RAC) that address trials for gene therapy. Phase I trials are considered safety trials and use only a small number—from 2 to 20—of adult subjects who are fully informed about the nature of the test. The FDA carefully reviews the data in the investigational new drug (IND) application, looking especially for adverse events.
Phase II	If the drug appears safe in humans, investigators recruit a large number of subjects—from 100 to 300—to continue safety studies and evaluate how well the drug works. Researchers carefully record all the data; the FDA closely monitors the study, again looking for adverse events and whether the drug is doing what it is supposed to do. This procedure is very time-consuming and costly. Many studies are discontinued at this stage.
Phase III	In this phase investigators recruit thousands of people from a variety of population centers. A new entity emerging worldwide in the enterprise of research is the contract research organization (CRO), which recruits subjects to participate in trials and conducts the day-to-day administration of research. Massive amounts of data are collected before presenting a new drug application (NDA) to the FDA. If the results of the trials are accepted by the FDA the drug is approved for marketing.
Phase IV	After approval, the drug's performance is monitored for long-term effects in a follow-up that may take from 10 to 20 months. The FDA may pull the drug from the market if problems arise.

[1]Most gene therapy trials in the United States are currently in the preclinical stage; a few have advanced to Phase I.

Source: Developed by Evelyn B. Kelly.

Safety and Animal Models of Disease

Judgments of the safety of gene therapy are based on animal data as compared to similar human interventions. Principles of disease pathogenesis and the development of gene therapy approaches can often be addressed by studying animal models of human disease. Animal models of genetic diseases have arisen spontaneously in a variety of species, including the mouse, cat, and dog. Using new methods to mutate genes in embryonic **stem cells,** scientists have engineered the alteration of any given gene in mice. For example, mouse mutations have exhibited a phenotype similar to the chronic granulomatous disease, hemophilia A, and spinocerebellar ataxia that are found in humans.

Unfortunately, animal models do not completely mimic human conditions. For example, the **CFTR gene** that is related to cystic fibrosis does not have the same pulmonary effects in animals as in humans. However, studying animal models has been a great boon for the advancement of gene therapy and other pharmacologic approaches. Feasibility and preclinical studies are done with animal models. Then, if a procedure appears promising, a research company or educational institution may implement a plan for testing in several stages:

- Feasibility testing, which involves studies and in vitro experiments on human cells, but not with patients.
- Early clinical research, which involves a few human subjects with rare and severe disease for whom other treatment alternatives are too risky, not applicable, or less likely to provide benefit.
- Clinical testing, which occurs only if potential success has been shown in earlier trials. This stage of testing may involve a wider range of diseases and more patients.

Some genetic diseases, such as the blood disorder thalassemia, have counterparts in animals. For other diseases, making judgments about the safety of data based on animals could provide basic information, although the clinical benefit from the study of disease in these animals cannot be measured.

Questions of safety include not only short-term effects, but also long-term consequences that may require years to determine—even in animals. Long-term studies of generations of animals may also be required if germ-line therapy is ever anticipated. The next section discusses factors to consider before deciding to follow a gene therapy protocol.

Efficacy

Research must show that the procedure will work. Evidence must be provided that the proposed therapy will deliver a gene to a tissue where it is effective. The gene must remain in the cells long enough to have an effect and the desired product must be observed.

Reliability

Procedures must demonstrate that the clinical benefits outweigh the risks of ill effects or failure.

Table 2-2 Phases of Gene Therapy in Trials Worldwide

Phase	Number of Gene Therapy Trials
I	743
I and II	242
II	169
II and III	12
III	26
Total	1192

Adapted by Evelyn B. Kelly from *The Journal of Gene Medicine,* updated July 2006.

Alternative Treatments

Gene therapy is acceptable only if it has the best prospect of success from among all other possible treatments. Drugs can treat some genetic effects.

Severity of Symptoms

Persons afflicted with some diseases have such dim prospects for quality of life that the family may determine that the risks of treatment are preferable to living with the disease. For example, a person with the genetic **Lesch–Nyhan disease** has such poor prospects for quality of life that the patient may decide that the risk of gene therapy is preferable to letting the condition run its natural course.

Informed Consent

This is a most important consideration in gene therapy (discussed in more depth in Chapter 9). A person who is a candidate for gene therapy must be made aware of the possible risks of mutation, the possible effects on the germ line and other side effects, and the relative costs, risks, and benefits of alternative therapies.

A number of methods have been used and are currently being invented for the efficient and safe delivery of therapeutic DNA. Yet the increasing variety of methods indicates that there is no single clearly ideal delivery system. Although clinical trials have begun, numerous limitations must be overcome before routine clinical care will be possible. The trials for approval of drugs and gene therapy procedures are highly rigidly overseen. At present, the U.S. Food and Drug Administration (FDA) has not approved any procedure for gene therapy.

In summation, the development of new approaches to gene therapy requires a staff of specialists to support and gain approval for the research and to analyze results. From beginning to end, it is a time-consuming process, as outlined below:

- Researchers learn all they can about a disease, determine whether it is a good candidate for gene therapy, secure funding for the project, and then design preclinical animal studies.
- Using their knowledge about the disorder, researchers design the therapy and then test it in appropriate models.

- Researchers now obtain financial support and approval for trials.
- For Phase I trials, researchers recruit a small group of people willing to test the safety and dosage limits of the proposed therapy. It takes time to evaluate the results before going to the next step.
- For Phase II trials, researchers recruit 100 to 300 people who continue to test the safety and efficacy of the therapy and evaluate how well it is working. Analysis of the results is time consuming.
- For Phase III trials, researchers enlist 1,000 to 3,000 people to test the effectiveness of the therapy.
- To gain FDA approval, researchers write proposals, complete paper work, and answer questions. One FDA regulator commented at a meeting that semitrucks have been seen backing in to deliver the documents. Some researchers are hoping that a new electronic system will streamline the approval process.
- Researchers then wait for FDA approval. If approval is granted, Phase IV trials continue to monitor the procedure for 10 to 20 months, when it may become available for general use.

The procedure outlined above explains why the development of new approaches to gene therapy is so time consuming. For example, the concept of using gene therapy for adenosine deaminase (ADA) was conceived more than 30 years ago, with trials beginning in earnest about 15 years ago—and still, no procedure has succeeded in being approved for use in common medical practice. Although challenges continue to persist, the technology and techniques of gene therapy are continuing to improve.

CHAPTER 3

Discoveries Leading to Gene Therapy

During the sixteenth and seventeenth centuries, doctors touted urine as liquid gold. In their bottles, these *piss prophets* were scrutinized, swirled, and even tasted for clues about what was wrong inside the body. Reading urine also became a popular way of telling fortunes—usually by predicting that the liquid's donor would come into a great sum of money. In the eighteen and nineteenth centuries, the scams gave way to scientific investigation and the important work of chemist Alexander Garrod (1857–1936).

The British physician Alexander Garrod was interested in colors, and the colored pigments in urine fascinated him. At the Great Osmond Street Hospital for Children, he was called to visit 3-month-old Thomas P., whose urine was a deep reddish brown. He diagnosed the boy as having alkaptonuria, a rare condition in which a type of acid, alkapton, builds up in the body. Normally, the acid is broken down, but in rare cases the acid is excreted in the urine and turns black when exposed to air. Garrod studied members of the boy's family and found that relatives had inter-married. When he learned that a fifth child had been born with the same condition, it occurred to him that the disease might be inherited. Mendel's work had just been discovered in England, and Garrod suspected that this condition fit the recessive characteristics that Mendel had written about in his *PEAS*. Garrod established a new class of diseases called "inborn errors of metabolism"—hereditary diseases—not based on bacteria, but on inheritance. However, it was not until the 1940s, several years after his death, that Garrod's work was applied to gene theory. Garrod's understanding of the inborn errors of body chemistry laid the foundation for the idea that changing the inborn error might some day be possible: thus was conceived the idea of gene therapy.

From the time that human beings could reason, they realized that there must be some mechanism of passing characteristics from one generation to another. They noted how the chin or nose of a parent was present in offspring. Also, they began to connect certain illnesses or diseases as being passed down. For example, ancient Jews recognized hemophilia or the bleeding disease. The Talmud excused newborn boys from circumcision when a mother had lost several sons to uncontrolled bleeding as a result of this ceremony. These people realized that certain characteristics were passed from mother to son—although knowledge of the blood-clotting gene for Factor VIII was unknown.

History has mixed evaluations about tampering with fate. The utopian dream to eliminate disease has captivated humankind for many eons. Television specials such as "Making Perfect People" or similarly themed magazine articles draw large viewing audiences and have huge newsstand sales. Although people are interested in speculation about the future of gene therapy, they also fear the possibilities. Novels such as *Brave New World* showed genetic engineering as a slippery slope to manipulating human beings at the beckoning of the government. In the hands of greedy people, evil may emerge. Yet the potential for good is also there, and scientists know that they have grave responsibility. This chapter considers the historical background of the development of gene therapy through the 1980s. Topics that lay this foundation include the dreams and efforts of ancient humans, the eugenics movement, human genetic development and the genome, the identification of amino acids, and genetic engineering.

DREAMS OF PERFECT PEOPLE

As early as 5000 BC, some societies demonstrated an understanding of inheritance. Humans began to breed selectively hardy varieties of livestock and crops, such as wheat, maize, and dates. Aristotle pondered how traits can be passed to offspring and developed sophisticated ideas, such as that injuries sustained in life could be passed on to offspring. His theory of **pangenesis** attempted to explain how traits are passed through particles called *gemules* to the mother.

For thousands of years people have tried to rank each other according to perceived superiority or inferiority. The Greek philosopher Socrates (470–399 BC) suggested that some people were born to lead, some to follow, and others to work. The idea of a perfect world emerged among the Greeks when Aristophanes, in *The Birds,* described a city in the clouds whose citizens were superior to the worldly Athenians. In *The Republic* Plato invented a complete community in which the natural rulers were the philosophers, followed by the warriors and the workers, who were assigned social roles based on their abilities. In the Middle Ages people were grouped as rulers, aristocracy, and peasants. Talents and intelligence were obviously recognized to be unequally distributed among people. Certain traits such as musical or mathematical ability, intelligence, and criminality, appeared to run in families.

In the sixteenth century, Sir Thomas More named his book *Utopia,* describing a place where ideals of working and community led to harmony and happiness. The term *utopia* has come to mean an ideal place of peace. Nearly 150 utopian communities existed in the United States, including Brook Farm in Massachusetts and the Oneida Community in New York. But the movement was soon overtaken by a new ideology, Darwinism. When Charles Darwin (1809–1882), a proponent of Aristotle's idea of pangenesis, published his *Origin of Species* in 1859, some thinkers began to apply the principles of natural selection to people as groups, or even to entire races. According to Social Darwinism, weak members of society would be unable to compete and survive, so they and their culture must be destroyed. Using this logic, millionaires were the fittest members of society.

One of the first to write about and promote racial superiority was Arthur de Gobineau (1816–1882) in his 1856 book *The Inequality of the Races.* He promoted the superiority of the Aryan or German race. The German philosopher Ernst Haeckle (1834–1919) embraced this idea and promoted breeding among the Nordic races. Friedrich Nietzsche wrote about the *Ubermenschen* [supermen] in a society filled with ideal people. Herbert Spencer (1820–1893) was an English eugenicist who believed, along with the mathematician Thomas Malthus (1766–1834), that there would be soon too many people on the earth for it to sustain life and that only the fittest would survive.

All these speculations culminated in the *eugenics* movement, a term coined by Francis Galton, British scientist and cousin of Darwin, in 1882. The term is based on the Greek word *eugenes,* meaning "good in birth." **Eugenics** is the practice of attempting to improve the human race by selective breeding. The rationale is to remove bad genes from the population, thus increasing the genetic fitness of humanity as a result. In the United States between 1911 and 1930, 24 states passed laws that restricted—either by requiring sterilization or by prohibiting marriage—the right of the "unfit" to have children. In the early decades of the twentieth century, the principles of eugenics were embraced in Germany, especially after the Nazi party's rise to power in 1933; the architects of the Holocaust sought to exterminate Jews and others who were considered inferior.

The philosophy of eugenics still holds currency to a minor degree in modern society. For example, some people think that genetic engineering can create a superior race. Based on genetic screening, a couple might decide not to have children or to terminate a pregnancy. In 1994 China imposed restrictions on marriage by individuals with certain disabilities and diseases.

However, people began to realize that eugenics as a theory had no advantages in a caring, progressive society. There is evidence that it could never be effective: calculations of the frequency of deleterious alleles in the population show that at least 1 percent of the genes carry something that could be fatal. Even if scientists predicted the effects that might be achieved by preventing all people with a given gene from producing offspring, the effect would be minimal.

When the emergence of biotechnology, with terms such as *recombinant DNA* (rDNA), hit the newspapers, the public recalled the horrific experiments of the Nazis and the philosophy of the eugenicists. The memory of Nazi pograms haunted the development of genetic engineering in the 1970s. People became frightened at the proposition of changing genes, whether to heal a lethal gene or to enhance some personal characteristic such as intelligence.

GENETICS DEVELOPMENT AND THE HUMAN GENOME

In 1866 Gregor Mendel (1822–1884), an Austrian monk living in a monastery in Brunn, published a report showing that characteristics of an organism were inherited. A Swiss scientist, Friedrich Miescher, who was only 25 years old at the time, purified DNA in 1869. He initially isolated the material, which he called *nuclein,* from white blood cells in pus. By August 1869, he had isolated that same material from yeast, kidney, liver, testes, and nucleated red blood cells: the material proved to be DNA. It is a curious twist of fate that two men, Mendel and Miescher, in a time span of only three years and living only a few hundred miles apart, would both make key discoveries that lay the foundation of modern molecular biology and that both works would be sorely neglected. In 1882 the German biologist Walter Fleming (1843–1905) discovered chromosomes and named them after two Greek root words, *chromos,* meaning "color," and *soma,* meaning "body." The bodies appeared colored when they were stained with dye. In the 1890s German geneticist Albrecht Kossel (1853–1927) pointed to the role of DNA in heredity. However, the work of these early scientists was forgotten for the rest of the nineteenth century.

In the early twentieth century, scientists rediscovered the work of Mendel and Miescher. In 1900 cell biologists in Germany and the United States independently observed the link between Mendel's units of inheritance and the chromosomes. In 1905 biologist William Bateson first used the term *genetics.*

In 1906 Thomas Hunt Morgan and colleagues at Columbia University began studying heredity in the fruit fly (drosophila). By 1912 Morgan's colleague, American geneticist A. H. Sturtevant (1891–1970), constructed the first chromosome map, which showed that genes for specific traits could be mapped to their locations on the four fruit fly chromosomes. These early geneticists likened their work to that in the famous parable of the blind man who feels the shape and contours of an elephant. But they had discovered that the gene had a concrete physical reference point on the chromosome.

Some scientists in the 1920s sought a more specific description of the gene by looking at its molecular composition. One of Miescher's students, Richard Altman, suggested a new name for Miescher's nuclein: nucleic acids. In 1925 studies began to show that X-rays induced mutations in genetic materials.

A turning point came in 1928 when Frederick Griffith discovered that the nonvirulent R type of the virus *pneumococcus* could be turned into the deadly S type. He found that heating the S type to kill the bacteria and then mixing it with the living, nonlethal R type changed it into its deadly cousin. Griffith had no idea that the DNA material from S was getting into R and changing it genetically. Unfortunately, he and his experiments were lost when his London laboratory was bombed during World War II. However, in New York City, Oswald Avery (1877–1955) at Rockefeller University heard of Griffith's results, but he did not believe them. He and his colleagues set out to discover what made one strain of pneumococcus change to another strain. They carefully separated protein from sugar and fats from nucleic acid and concluded that only the nucleic acid transformed the cells. When they published their results in the *Journal of Experimental Biology* in 1944, they received a cool reception from other biologists. The thinking at the time was that proteins—not DNA—carried the genes or units of heredity.

In 1952 two scientists at Cold Spring Harbor Laboratory presented evidence that Avery and colleagues were correct. Alfred Hershey and Martha Chase showed how viruses that attack bacteria only inject DNA into the host cell and that no protein enters the bacteria. The DNA from the virus directed the production of new viruses.

Avery had shown that changing genes was a possibility. While working at the University of Texas, Hermann Muller became one of the first to deliberately change genes by use of radiation. He was awarded the Nobel Prize in Physics or Medicine in 1946, but his work pointed only to random change in DNA and was therefore not useful for directed genetic change for a specific purpose such as gene therapy.

As more and more evidence accumulated that DNA was the genetic element, a small group of scientists in the 1940s and 1950s began to ask how a molecule such as DNA could carry genetic information. An unusual pair of scientists resolved this question. James Watson (1928–), a 24-year-old American geneticist, and Francis Crick (1916–2004), a British physicist, met at the Cavendish Laboratories in Cambridge in 1951. They were both convinced that the structure of DNA held the key to knowledge of how genetic information is stored and transmitted to daughter cells. A technique known as *X-ray crystallography* revealed the answer to the question. When X-rays are directed at a crystal of some material, atoms in the substance refract and reflect. A trained observer studying the X-ray pattern can see pictures of the molecule. Maurice Wilkins and Rosalind Franklin of Kings College had taken pictures of DNA in 1951, but they did not recognize what they were seeing. Watson saw their picture and rushed back to Cambridge to convince Crick to make an all-out effort to construct the molecule. They worked continuously for a week and made a Tinkertoy-like molecule, shifting atoms to match the X-ray photograph. They built a model consisting of two helices, or corkscrew spirals, that wrapped around each other. Each helix had a backbone of alternating sugar and phosphate groups, and to each sugar was attached one of four nitrogen bases: adenine, thymine, cytosine, and guanine. The sugar phosphate formed the sides of the ladder, or backbone, and the nitrogen bases appeared like rungs on the ladder. They were not arranged at random, but A always joined to T, and C always joined to G. The scientists revealed their model on March 7, 1953, and won the 1954 Nobel Prize in Chemistry. They even began to surmise the role of DNA in the manufacture of proteins in the cell.

After the discovery of the structure of DNA, Marshall Nirenberg (1927–) announced in 1961 that he had discovered the process for unraveling the code of DNA. His research involved the genetic code sequences for amino acids, the building blocks of proteins. He found the specific sequences or patterns that code for 20 amino acids. This study paved the way for understanding genetic diseases and later to the idea of controlling hereditary units. Also, in this same year, Francis Crick and South African geneticist Sydney Brenner reported that triplets of DNA bases, called *nucleotides,* program the 20 amino acids that make up proteins.

Rollin D. Hotchkiss, a colleague of Avery's, began to think about transferring genes to mammalian cells. Beginning in the 1950s, he sought to transfer a mouse pigmented strain to nonpigmented embryos. But things did not go well for him, and he never found one transformed mouse cell. However, in a talk in 1965, he was the first to coin the term *genetic engineering.*

In 1956 Joshua Lederberg and colleagues at Rockefeller University discovered that, when viruses infect bacterial cells, bits of DNA from the host chromosome are incorporated into the offspring of the new viruses. The viruses can then infect new bacteria and deposit in them the bacterial genes that the viruses have picked up elsewhere. These new host cells can become permanently changed by incorporating the genes into their own genomes. This discovery suggested that viruses could be used to transfer genes into other cells; however, transfer of genes for therapeutic purposes would involve getting the desired genes into eukaryotic cells.

An unusual early gene therapy treatment resulted from a study of warts on laboratory workers at Oak Ridge National Laboratory in Tennessee. Dr. Stanfield Rogers had been studying a virus that caused hornlike warts on wild rabbits. He found that the blood of the workers had high levels of the amino acid arginine; the virus carried the gene to make arginase, an enzyme that breaks down arginine. The workers had no ill effects because the virus was transferring arginase to them, like having an agent for therapy without a disease. Then in 1969 Lederberg read of two German girls who had high levels of arginine in their blood, prohibiting their bodies from producing urea. Consequently, the by-product of ammonia built up and caused the girls to become epileptic and grossly retarded. Rogers purified the virus and took it to Cologne, Germany, where he treated the girls. The treatments were not really effective, and Rogers found himself at the center of an ethical controversy. Yet in 1971 he was the first to attempt human gene therapy, in a historical but unappreciated experiment that put gene therapy on the map.

In 1971 Carl R. Merrill, a researcher at the National Institutes of Health (NIH), described in *Nature* how he had infected human fibroblasts growing in a culture with a *lambda* virus that was carrying an *Escherichia coli* gene. He reasoned that the next step would be to consider viruses for their ability to transfer genes to cells.

The genetic engineering revolution dawned in 1972 when respected scientist Ernst Freese convened a meeting at NIH's Stone House headquarters. The meeting brought together leading researchers representing the many areas of work being conducted in the field of gene therapy, and sought to develop ethical guidelines.

AMINO ACIDS DISCOVERED

Chapter 1 emphasized how amino acids are the building blocks of proteins programmed by genes. Understanding how proteins and genes are interrelated was essential in the development of gene therapy.

The nineteenth century proved to be a great age for the beginnings of chemistry. The first few amino acids were discovered in the early 1800s. In 1806 Louis Nicolas Vauquelin isolated aspargine from asparagus. In 1812 William Hyde Wollaston found that urine, the darling of the *piss prophets* of the eighteenth century, contained a second amino acid. In 1820 Henri Braconnot, a French chemist, discovered two natural amino acids, glycine and cystine. Around the end of the century, arginine, histidine, and lysine were found, although the scientists did not know the relationship between amino acids and protein molecules. In 1899 German scientist

Emil Fischer synthesized many of the 13 amino acids known at that time and found three more. He also showed how these amino acids combined with each other inside the protein molecule. He even suggested that combinations of these chains of amino acids help establish the characteristics of different proteins. Some scientists even surmised that these amino acids might be related to nutrition.

By the turn of the century, things began to change. Investigators were beginning to use the scientific method. In 1901 British biochemist Frederick Gowland Hopkins found that the amino acid tryptophan played an important role in the diet. He fed a group of mice only corn that contained the protein zein but no tryptophan; the mice did not thrive. Only when he added tryptophan-rich casein to the diet did the mice survive. In 1922 two other investigators found that tryptophan and lysine were essential for normal growth in rats. In the 1930s American biochemist William C. Rose isolated threonine, the last of the nutritionally important amino acids. In humans, the essential amino acids are isoleucine, leucine, lysine, methionine, phenylalanine, threonine, tryptophan, valine, and in growing children histidine. Without these, the body does not have the building blocks to form new protein molecules and growth is impaired. All of these amino acids can be obtained from meats, eggs, milk, cheese, and other foods derived from animals; plant proteins lack several of the amino acids and must be supplemented.

The studies of inherited metabolic conditions provided another approach to the biochemical mechanisms of genes. George Wells Beadle (1903–1989) and Edward Lawrie Tatum (1909–1975) established the *one-gene-one enzyme* theory through their studies of *Neurospora crassa,* the red bread mold. Building on the previous work of Alexander Garrod and Linus Pauling (1901–1994), who established the molecular basis of sickle cell anemia, Beadle and Tatum sealed the relationship between genes and enzymes.

THE BIRTH OF GENETIC ENGINEERING

The exact beginning of genetic engineering is difficult to determine. Genetic engineering, or rDNA technology, uses the techniques of molecular biology to alter the genome of an organism. For example, inserting exogenous DNA from the outside of the cell alters the genome of the receiving organism. Discovering genetic material and the technical means to manipulate this material opened up a new era of genetic technology.

The discovery of **restriction enzymes** was an important step. Scientists found that some viruses not only attack people, but can also be the scourge of the microbial world. Called **bacteriophages**—literally, bacteria eaters—these viruses are simple pieces of DNA that attach to the bacterium and inject their own DNA into the cell. When the phage gets inside the cell, it takes over and forces the host to make more viral DNA and protein. Then the cell ruptures, and a new generation of viruses is released. Some bacteria protect themselves from these phages by producing enzymes that cut foreign DNA into shorter pieces: these enzymes that cut or restrict the viruses are called restriction enzymes. In 1970 Hamilton O. Smith, a scientist at Johns Hopkins University, discovered the first restriction enzyme, called *Hind*III, which searches the DNA for the sequence

AAGCT and cuts the chain between the two A's. Smith shared a Nobel Prize with two others for this discovery.

The first restriction enzyme led to a vast array of enzymes from many bacteria, with each one cutting at a specific point. For example, the enzyme *Eco*R1 recognizes the sequence GAATTC and cuts between the G and A. Finding this enzyme led to another great discovery of genetic engineering—the ability to put two different pieces of DNA together. Also, in the early 1970s, Paul Berg (1926–) at Stanford University isolated DNA from the bacterium *Escherichia coli* and a virus from a monkey, SV40. By cutting both samples with *Eco*R1 and mixing them together, he made the first hybrid molecule in the test tube. This recombining—splicing two sources together—became known as *rDNA*. This became the foundation for the modern sciences of biotechnology and, ultimately, gene therapy. Berg was awarded a Nobel Prize in 1980 for this important discovery.

Plasmids are small, circular pieces of DNA bacteria that are separate from the normal chromosomal DNA of the bacterium. In the 1970s Stanley Cohen and Herbert Boyer, at Stanford, found that, if they cut plasmids from different sources using *Eco*R1, the two plasmid pieces would stick together. They also discovered that a piece of DNA from the chromosome of another organism—cut with the same enzyme—forms that hybrid. Once inside the cell, the plasmid and its new material replicates normally as the bacteria divides. When the bacteria divide, millions of copies are made in a process called *gene cloning*.

How can scientists determine the location of the desired DNA? Cohen and Boyer found that by using a plasmid that contains two different antibiotic-resistant genes—one for ampicillin resistance, *ampR,* and one for tetracycline resistance, *tetR*—they could create marker genes. A **genetic marker** is a particular gene or DNA base sequence that is associated with a particular chromosome. These markers are associated with particular genes or traits. For example, scientists have found genetic markers associated with traits found in patients with risk factors for heart disease and asthma as well as other diseases.

Genetic markers have three essential properties:

- They are easily identifiable.
- They are associated with a specific locus on a chromosome.
- They are **polymorphic,** meaning they must have two or more distinct forms that exist within a single breeding population of a species.

The history of the idea of changing genes developed slowly and painfully. At a symposium called "Reflection on Research and the Future of Medicine" in 1966, Josua Lederberg and Edward Tatum laid out the fundamental ideas that became gene therapy:

- Restriction enzymes allow scientists to cut DNA in specific locations and to insert new DNA to make rDNA. That new DNA could be a gene.
- Plasmids provide a vector for putting new DNA into another organism.
- Marker genes enable screening of a culture and selection for cells that have been transformed with rDNA.

EARLY ATTEMPTS AT GENE THERAPY

Between 1970 and 1973, Dr. Stanfield Rogers, an American, and a German physician attempted to treat three girls with **arginemia,** a debilitating genetic disease, by administering the Shope papilloma virus that the physicians believed might supplement the missing enzyme gene argininase. The treatment was unsuccessful. These experiments were performed before ethics review boards, and were discussed openly. After the trials, a discussion centered on whether there was enough evidence to anticipate that the girls would benefit. The ethical debate about the Shope virus experiments is still unresolved, although, clearly, no legal or institutional precepts were violated.

CONTROVERSIAL CLINE

In 1980 Martin Cline, an American scientist and physician at the University of California Los Angeles (UCLA), became the first investigator to attempt gene therapy using rDNA. The treatments were carried out in Israel and Italy on two patients with beta-thalassemia. Cline took bone marrow samples from each patient, treated them with DNA containing a normal hemoglobin protein gene, and then returned the treated bone marrow cells. To accomplish this, he had to kill a portion of the patients' native cells by radiation. At the time of the experiment, Cline's request for review was pending. He conducted the experiments on July 10 and 15, and the UCLA Human Subject Protection Committee disapproved of the proposal on July 16. There was no debate: the consensus was that Cline's experiments had been premature and unethical. Cline resigned his position and lost his NIH grants. The issues raised by his controversial experiments pointed out the importance of federal research policy decisions. Cline's actions were in direct violation of NIH gene therapy guidelines and were taken without the approval of the Institutional Review Board at UCLA. Ethical concerns caused a number of groups—including the National Council of Churches, the Synagogue Council of America, and the United States Catholic Conference—to ask for a review. The NIH censured Cline for conducting an rDNA experiment. These trials led to the formation of committees charged with exploring the ethics of gene therapy and human experimentation.

Although gene therapy presented hope, several failed genetic experiments led to caution and questions. However, in the 1990s, with the advent of the Human Genome Project and advances in genetic technology, the vision of using genes for therapy developed into more than just a good idea.

CHAPTER 4

Successes and Setbacks in the 1990s

French Anderson, an undergraduate student at Harvard, was excited when he transferred genes from one bacterium into another in his laboratory experiments. He often lay awake at night, wondering if it would be possible to cure human disease in this way. At a seminar one day, a professor presented the latest research on the genetic makeup of hemoglobin. Raising his hand, Anderson questioned the possibility of putting a gene for normal hemoglobin into a patient with sickle cell anemia. The professor snapped at him and informed the inquisitive undergraduate that this was a serious discussion with no room for foolish statements. Deflated, Anderson sank into silence. After the meeting another professor came up to him and expressed interest in the question he had asked. In their biography, *W. French Anderson: Father of Gene Therapy* (2003), Bob Burke and Barry Epperson recount how this interesting idea became an obsession for the student, who decided on that day in 1958 that this would be his calling: human gene therapy.

Although the Nazi experiments and failed eugenics policies still haunted the thinking of some people, the attitude in the decades of the 1970s and 1980s was basically that the science of medicine would solve just about all problems. After all, in the public's perception, marvelous and powerful antibiotics were wiping out all bacterial diseases. Science could conquer all diseases, even those with genetic causes. According to a 1992 poll conducted by Louis Harris and Associates for the March of Dimes, 87 percent of U.S. adults were willing to use gene transfer technology to cure a fatal disease. That was the attitude at the beginning of the last decade of the twentieth century.

Several pivotal events affected hopes for genetic medicine in the 1990s:

- The favorable outcome of the Human Genome Project (HGP)
- The first successful gene therapy project
- The discovery of genes that cause various disorders
- A failed experiment that got lots of press

By the end of the twentieth century, gene therapy, which had started out with high expectations at the beginning of the decade, had become a questionable science struggling to climb its way back to respectability.

THE HUMAN GENOME PROJECT: BORN IN 1990

The Human Genome Project (HGP) was a massive scientific effort to identify all of the human genes and to determine the sequence of the chemical bases— adenine, thymine, cytosine, guanine—of the human genome. At the time the genome was thought to have 50,000 to 100,000 genes, constructed from 3 billion base pairs of nucleotides located on 23 pairs of chromosomes.

The idea of completing the genome sequence first came from an unexpected source, the U.S. Department of Energy. Fearing attacks with nuclear weapons, the department was concerned with measuring the mutation rate of human DNA exposed to low-level radiation. At a meeting in 1984 in Alta, Utah, department leaders suggested sequencing the genome as a way to measure the effects of radiation. A second impetus came from health professionals who thought that the project could lead to the treatment of a large variety of genetic illnesses. In 1987 the discovery of the gene that caused cystic fibrosis fueled excitement in the medical community to identify other genes. The HGP would provide possibilities for conquering human disease.

In 1987 the Department of Energy's Biological and Environmental Research Advisory Committee (RAC) recommended the large-scale project to map the entire genome, with a target date of 2005. The HGP officially began in 1990, with James Watson, co-discoverer of the double helix in 1953, as the first director. When he resigned in 1992, Francis Collins, a leading genetics researcher at the University of Michigan, took over leadership of the project.

The actual gene sequencing was carried on in research centers in the United States, Japan, England, Germany, and China—with teams working on segments of chromosomes. However, the majority of the work was carried out at five institutions:

- The Whitehead Institute for Medical Research in Massachusetts
- Baylor College of Medicine in Texas
- The University of Washington
- The Joint Genome Institute in California
- The Sanger Center (near Cambridge) in the United Kingdom

In 1995 *Haemophilus influenzae,* the bacterium that causes influenza, became the first genome of an organism other than a virus to be sequenced. Producing such physical maps involves cutting DNA molecules using restriction enzymes, cloning (i.e., copying) the fragments, and finding overlapping fragments to analyze.

Another player soon entered the game. J. Craig Venter, a researcher at NIH, announced his revolutionary method for simultaneously identifying thousands of genes expressed in different tissues of the human body. With the help of the first commercially available DNA sequencer, Venter's laboratory could produce data on many genes, whereas others could study only one gene at a time. This process enabled him to bypass the 95 percent of the genome that apparently had no function, called *junk DNA*. In 1995 Venter formed a new company, Celera, that would complete sequencing of the human genome years ahead of the 2005 deadline.

In June 2000 President Clinton proudly stood beside Collins and Venter at the White House and declared that a rough draft of the genome had been completed well ahead of the target date. For development of the HGP since the announcement in 2000, see Chapter 13, Future of Gene Therapy.

W. FRENCH ANDERSON: FATHER OF GENE THERAPY

W. French Anderson was born in 1936 in Tulsa, Oklahoma, and entered Harvard in 1953, the same year that Watson and Crick unlocked the structure of DNA. The idea of supplanting defective genes with healthy genes was born in his mind in March 1958. Five years later, researchers Joshua Lederberg and Edward Tatum suggested that gene therapy held a future in medicine. Anderson came to NIH in 1965 and began to work on synthesizing hemoglobin, the red pigment that carries oxygen to the body cells. He focused on the blood and became well known for his work with thalassemia and sickle cell disease.

In the meantime, gene-splicing techniques were developed, and Anderson turned his attention in the 1970s to his original goal, dealing with disease at the molecular level. He was especially interested in ways of transferring engineered genes into cells. He found that using a needle to inject the genes was too limiting and impractical. Some other colleagues had toyed with the idea that the most efficient vector might be a virus, a simple organism that gets into the cell and takes over its genetic works. One type of virus in particular—the retrovirus—acts like a Trojan horse, sneaking genes into cells.

In the early 1980s techniques for stripping viruses of their harmful genetic material and techniques for cloning had been developed, and the retrovirus appeared to be a serious potential vector. Anderson was first interested in thalassemia but thought that the disease might be too complex for his present experiment, so he turned his attention to another hereditary disease, adenosine deaminase (ADA) deficiency, a condition in which an enzyme necessary for immune system function is missing. A single gene is responsible.

In 1984 the ADA gene was cloned at the University of Cincinnati. Two of three pieces of the puzzle were solved; the third piece was to locate the cells in which to insert the gene. Anderson identified the white blood cell—the T cell—as the target and, in a 1988 trial, successfully placed genetically tagged cells into terminal cancer patients. He found these cells would reproduce inside the body.

However, in the 1980s publicity about manipulation of human genes led to an outpouring of ethical and political concern. Although Anderson became discouraged, he continued working; the Congressional hearings concluded that gene

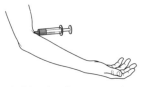

1. Blood cells removed
   from patient

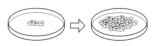

2. Specialized white blood cells,
   called T cells, are grown in
   laboratory cultures.

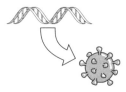

3. Normal ADA genes are
   inserted into specially
   engineered viruses.

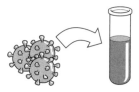

4. Viruses are mixed with the
   T cells, infecting the cells and
   allowing the ADA genes to be
   spliced into the cells
   chromosomes

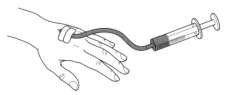

5. The patient receives an injection
   of about a billion "infected" T cells.

Figure 4-1
Anderson's Gene Therapy Experiment.

therapy was neither unethical nor immoral if properly regulated. It took two years for the first human trials of gene therapy to take place. See Chapter 10, Regulation of Gene Therapy.

On March 30, 1990, Anderson and two other colleagues submitted a document of several hundred pages to the Human Gene Therapy Committee of the RAC, proposing to reprogram the genetic code of children suffering from ADA deficiency. The proposal seemed astounding:

1. The human ADA gene would be spliced into a mutant mouse retrovirus.
2. Blood taken from the patient would be exposed to the mouse virus.
3. After the cultured cells were enriched in a growth substance, they would be given back to the patient in a series of monthly injections.

In other words, Anderson and his colleagues proposed putting a healthy copy of a gene into the bone marrow cells of a sick person. The treated cells would then be injected into the child to produce the enzyme that could correct the defective one.

One member of the committee was Michael Hershfield, the scientist who created the drug PEG-ADA, which had succeeded in keeping children with ADA alive past the age of two. The drug links ADA to a molecule of polyethylene glycol (PEG), and supplies a normal copy of the enzyme to the patient. Treatment with PEG-ADA is a painful procedure in which patients are subjected to injections every other day for the rest of their lives. Also, PEG-ADA cost about $60,000 per year, and was really not a cure. Hershfield was concerned that gene therapy might endanger the progress the drug was making in treating the children.

Anderson informed the committee that he had chosen ADA because the disease had several of the features necessary for gene therapy. He also presented the potential risks. After several days' bureaucratic discussion, he was finally granted approval.

ASHANTHI'S STORY

Four-year-old Ashanthi DeSilva, or Ashi, was a charming little girl with raven-black hair and big brown eyes from North Olmstead, Ohio. Her parents, Raj and Van DeSilva, drove 400 miles to Bethesda to talk to W. French Anderson and Michael Blaese, the pediatrician involved in the gene therapy project. Ashi had taken PEG-ADA for several years, but the effect was failing. Her parents understood the risks that may be involved in gene therapy, but their little girl was dying. They signed the informed consent forms.

ADA is a form of genetic disorder called severe combined immuno-deficiency disease (SCID), which keeps the person who has it from fighting off other diseases, even mild ones like the common cold or influenza. Most children die before their second birthday. The ADA deficiency is traced to the long arm of chromosome 20 (see Chapter 5, Single-Gene Disorders).

As Anderson pushed Ashi's wheelchair into the operating room, the nurse brought in the vinyl bag filled with cells that would soon be in her bloodstream. The infusion took about 28 minutes. For the first time, a living person underwent the procedure to receive a healthy gene. Another little girl, 9-year-old Cindy Cutshall, was also treated. She had a milder form of ADA and showed only modest improvements. But Ashi's treatment was an overwhelming success.

Anderson became more famous than a rock star during the following days. Evening news broadcasters announced that the age of genetic treatments had arrived. The story made the front page of major newspapers. The publicity surrounding the two successful trials encouraged other scientists to begin human gene therapy. The days of gene therapy had arrived, and Anderson was kindly called "the father of gene therapy."

As for Ashi, she was really a smashing success. In the spring of 1991 the whole family came down with the flu. Ashi was the first one up and about, and was even running around. The family's immune-deficient daughter had become a healthy, normal child. In 2002, at age 15, Ashi was a normal teenager, playing the piano and performing with the school band.

The experiments showed that gene therapy could be used successfully to treat human disease, and served as the proof of principle on which more than 600 clinical protocols could be based. In 1991 a protocol to treat malignant melanoma was approved. Other programs began in centers in the United States such as St. Jude's Children's Research Hospital in Memphis, Tennessee; the University of Wisconsin; the University of Pittsburgh; and in Italy, France, Canada, and the Netherlands.

WAS THIS A BRAVE NEW WORLD?

In 1932 Aldous Huxley wrote a novel, *Brave New World,* in which embryos are engineered to become leaders, followers, and menial laborers. The book agitated restless currents of distrust about science. When Watson and Crick announced the DNA model in 1953, the debate heated up again. The phrase "brave new world" was applied to prospects about genetics in which people feared that the manipulation of genes would be aimed at unethical attempts to create "perfect people." Again with the 1990 announcement of human gene therapy, critics began to charge that this procedure would lead to Huxley's vision. What could happen was impressed on the minds of people who argued that, as gene therapy became more refined and less expensive, it would be only a short step to tinkering with eye color, intelligence, or attention span.

Even professional colleagues attacked these treatments; at an international meeting, one scientist accused Anderson of seeking publicity and promoting bad science. But Anderson did not hesitate to let people know there was still an element of risk in gene therapy—he feared the worst if the public expected too much. Anderson's prescient words did not lessen the impact of what happened in 1999.

A MAJOR SETBACK

The gene therapy community was riding high during the 1990s, and failures were few. However, several trials to cure patients with SCID-ADA were unsuccessful, reducing the initial success rate to 1 in 20. Most scientists were not concerned with the low success rate, realizing that in such a novel procedure there would be wrinkles to iron out.

In 1995 at the University of Pennsylvania, Dr. James Wilson and Dr. Mark Batshaw joined the Institute for Human Gene Therapy (IHGT). Batshaw was interested in the genetic deficiency of a liver enzyme, ornithine transcarbamylase (OTC), which causes ammonia levels to build up in the blood. If left untreated, this chemical buildup causes convulsions, vomiting, coma, and death. Batshaw convinced Wilson that this condition should be the subject of their first gene therapy trial. Rather than use a retrovirus vector, they decided on an adenovirus (AD virus), which, in animal models, appeared to be more efficient. They worked out the details of the protocol and were granted a phase I gene therapy trial for adult patients with OTC deficiency.

The trial began in 1998 with 18 patients. One was 18-year-old Jesse Gelsinger from Arizona. On the second day of treatment, Jesse lapsed into a coma and died within 24 hours. The NIH immediately put a ban on all AD virus gene therapy trials and launched an investigation that lasted until 2001. However, Jesse's death also sounded the death knell for gene therapy and, certainly, for the careers of Wilson and Batshaw.

Gelsinger's death had the same effect on the gene therapy community that the Columbia space shuttle disaster had on NASA. However, both events brought attention to the need to prevent future accidents. The researchers had ignored warnings that could have prevented the death of Gelsinger and the illnesses of other participants in the trial. The FDA and the NIH initiated new stringent guidelines and safety regulations. See Chapter 10, Regulation of Gene Therapy.

THE FIRST GERM-LINE TRANSFER

People are more frightened of germ-line therapy. Gene therapy affecting these cells raised several concerns in addition to those of somatic cell therapy. Such therapy could be directed in several ways:

- Directly at the sperm or ova before the two unite at fertilization
- At the cells that produce the sperm or ova—precursor cells
- At the early stages of embryonic development, only hours after fertilization

Many religious traditions especially oppose germ-line experimentation. See Chapter 12, Social and Religious Issues. The major objections surrounding germ-line therapy concern the propagation of unpredictable effects into future generations and the long-term effects of changing genetic characteristics in human populations.

Genetic Treatment versus Eugenics

In a series of articles in *The New Yorker,* Daniel J. Kevles (1984) quoted Francis Galton as having defining eugenics as "the science [of] improving human stock by giving the more suitable races or strains of blood a better chance of prevailing over the less suitable." Gene therapy is defined as the medical intervention of replacing a defective gene that is not working with a healthy gene that is working.

Researchers are generally discreet about germ-line therapy, and getting approval for such protocols is extremely difficult. However, one type of germ-line therapy has been successful and has not caused controversy. As of 2001, 30 children were born as a result of transfer of the egg cytoplasm (ooplasm) performed on women who cannot conceive because of defects in their ooplasm. To correct the conditions, healthy ooplasm from donor eggs is injected into the defective eggs. A small amount of mitochondrial DNA is transferred into the egg, and the offspring has three genetic parents—with DNA from the mother, the father, and the ooplasm donor. This procedure is considered germ-line gene transfer because the DNA of these children and their offspring will always contain genetic material from all three parents.

As of July 2006, 1,192 gene therapy trials were ongoing worldwide. Although progress with a variety of diseases has been made in many areas, trials are proceeding with caution. Regulations in the United States and in other countries are strict and demanding. Chapters 5 through 8 discuss several initiatives in development.

The distinctions between gene therapy and eugenics are shown in Table 4-1.

Table 4-1   Gene Therapy versus Eugenics

Gene Therapy	Eugenics
Involves informed consent of patients who suffer from a specific disease	Involves social programs that are sometimes involuntary; focuses on general human traits
Intended to benefit a particular individual	Intended to improve humans in general or a national population
Directed at the correction of genes known to cause disease	Dwells on polygenic traits whose genetic composition is unknown or poorly understood
Involves genetic correction that does not affect the germ line and is like other medical procedures	Involves general goals that are not specifically intended for medical treatment

Created by Evelyn B. Kelly.

CHAPTER 5

Single-Gene Recessive Disorders

In September 2005 Ariel Coover lay on the operating room table at Cooper University Hospital in Camden, New Jersey, with only the top part of her bald head showing. Six catheters pumped 900 billion viral particles into her brain, along with a chance for a normal life. Ariel has Canavan disease, a degenerative neurological disease caused by a defect in a single recessive gene. The defect prevents the production of aspartoacylase, a brain enzyme that breaks down N-acetylaspartate acid into the elements needed to form myelin, the fatty covering of the nerve cells. The condition eventually causes the destruction of all of the myelin, followed by death.

Walter and Peggy Coover had another child named Amber who died of the disease. Their experience with Amber taught them a lot about the disease, and they learned that they were both carriers. The couple had one normal child, Dylan, but when Peggy became pregnant with Ariel, they found out through genetic screening that the fetus had the disease. They agonized for days about whether to have an abortion but decided not to go through this procedure. After Ariel's birth, they heard of the work at Cooper University Hospital and of neuroscientist Dr. Paola Leone, who was conducting a phase I study on patients with Canavan. Gene therapy does not cure the symptoms of Canavan, but it can stop them from progressing. Because Ariel was only three and a half months old, her parents hoped that early intervention would enable her to continue her development. For people like the Coovers, gene therapy offers hope that their children will be part of a miracle. Canavan is only one of many conditions that afflict people with genetic diseases.

Disease traits that are caused by genes may vary widely in their severity, depending on other genes and environmental factors. The term **expressivity** describes the extent to which a person has the signs or symptoms of the genetic disease. The term **penetrance** describes the expression of a gene in a population in which some people are affected and others who carry the gene are not affected. Complete penetrance indicates that everyone with the gene will have the disease; incomplete penetrance means that some people have the gene, but not the disease.

Genes can cause diseases through several mechanisms. Most diseases have both a genetic component inherited by the individual and an environmental component from outside the individual. The relative importance of heredity versus environment varies with the individual and with the disease. For example, medical conditions that are the result of war wounds or an automobile accident have little genetic input, but considerable environmental influences. Most diseases result from a mixture of genetics and environment; however, in a few diseases—such as Tay-Sachs disease and Huntington's disease—the genetic element is so strong that the disorders occur regardless of environment. Studying a particular family's "pedigree" can reveal whether the gene is **monogenic** (i.e., involving a single dominant or recessive gene), X-linked, or **polygenic** (i.e., involving many genes).

One of the first requirements for gene therapy to change mutant genes is to locate the gene that causes a specific disease. Chapters 5 through 8 discuss diseases and disorders caused by known genes. The chapters are arranged according to the inheritance pattern of the genes: single-gene recessive, single-gene dominant, X-linked disorders, and multiple genes. The section on each condition includes a description of the disease or condition, a brief history of the condition, and current efforts at targeting the mutant gene with gene therapy.

SINGLE-GENE RECESSIVE DISEASES

Single-gene recessive defects are those caused by mutations in one gene: they are monogenic. Mutations in DNA arise because of a spontaneous chemical change that results in a substitution, deletion, or insertion of a nucleotide base pair. Single-gene diseases contrast with those conditions and traits influenced by several genes or by environmental factors. Single-gene defects affect 1 to 2 percent of newborns.

SICKLE CELL DISEASE (SCD): PROTECTION AGAINST MALARIA

In the 1940s Anthony Allison, an Oxford graduate from Kenya, noted that the frequency of sickle cell disease (SCD) might be connected with the prevalence of malaria, a condition carried by mosquitoes. In 1949 Linus Pauling determined that SCD is caused by a defect in one of the genes that codes for hemoglobin. This mutation, which causes blood cells to collapse in the absence of oxygen, is frequently fatal to those who have two copies of the gene, but only mildly harmful to those with one copy. And those with one gene appear to be able to resist malaria. Allison tested the blood of Africans living in malarial areas and found that those with the sickle cells were less likely to have the malarial parasite. The mutation is common in parts of West Africa and is common in African Americans whose ancestors were brought to America as slaves. The disease also affects people of Mediterranean, Middle Eastern, and Indian ancestry. This very painful disease is a high price to pay today for malaria resistance in the past.

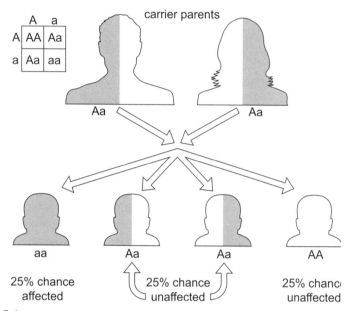

Figure 5-1
Single-gene carriers.

Sickle cell anemia is caused by a nucleotide base substitution, resulting in a defective hemoglobin molecule. Aberrant hemoglobin molecules constructed with these proteins have a tendency to stick to one another, forming strands of hemoglobin within the red blood cells. These strands elongate, making the blood cells stiff rather than round. The cells themselves thus appear sickle-shaped, hence the name.

Normal hemoglobin is composed of a *heme* molecule and two pairs of proteins called *globins*. Humans have genes to create six different types of globins: alpha, beta, gamma, delta, epsilon, and zeta. Which genes are expressed depends on whether the stage of development is embryonic, fetal, or adult. All hemoglobin produced in humans from the age of 2 to 3 months contains a pair of alpha-globin and beta-globin molecules.

SCD was the first genetic disorder known to point to a specific place where only one nucleotide is damaged. This site of the damage is called a **point mutation.** In the case of SCD, the mutation affects one nucleic acid along the entire strand of DNA that makes up the beta-globin gene. Specifically, thymine replaces adenine such that, when the amino acids are built, valine—GTG—takes the place of glutamic acid—GAG. Only one substitution creates a hemoglobin molecule that does not function normally.

Each person has two copies of the gene that makes beta-globin. SCD is an autosomal recessive disorder and results when the individual has two abnormal copies of the gene, one from each parent. One abnormal gene makes the person a carrier. The carrier does not normally have the symptoms of the condition, but an analysis of the blood may reveal some of the sickle cells. Approximately 2 million people worldwide carry the disease; 1 in 12 African Americans are carriers. About 1 in 500 African Americans and 1 in 1,000 Hispanic Americans have SCD.

In a study described in the 14 December 2001 edition of *Science,* Philippe Leboulch, a gene therapist, and a team of researchers at Harvard Medical School bioengineered mice to contain a human gene that produces the defective hemoglobin that causes SCD. Earlier studies showed that another protein, gamma-globin, keeps that cell from forming the sticky chains inside red blood cells, a process called polymerization. By adding part of the gamma-globin gene to a beta-globin gene, Leboulch's team found they could made hemoglobin that resists polymerization. Red blood cells arise from stem cells in the bone marrow. Leboulch's team took bone marrow from mice with SCD and added the modified gene to it. To deliver the genetic cargo to the mice, the team packaged modified beta-globin cells in a small piece of the human immunodeficiency virus (HIV) that infiltrated stem cells in the marrow. After 10 months nearly all of the red blood cells in the mice in the gene therapy group were making beta-globin coded by the engineered gene. Few sickle cells arose from the marrow stem cells. Leboulch agrees that this therapy is harsh, but, as a result of the success, he has planned future experiments in monkeys, a larger animal, in order to attempt to refine the process. A number of other studies are underway to produce less toxic regimens that would allow the new bone marrow to produce normal red blood cells in the long term.

Two years later, in 2003, Dana Levasseur and a team built on the previous work of correcting SCD in the mouse model, including three important additions:

1. They refined the mouse model and the lentivirus vector.
2. They provided direct evidence of the number of red cells expressing the transgene.
3. They addressed issues about the safety of gene therapy when the X-linked SCD cases developed a problem with the retrovirus insertions. The team transduced and transplanted only 1,000 enriched hematopoietic stems, which lessened the number of lentiviral integrations.

A successful application for treatment of human SCD is closer because of the work done with mouse models, but several issues must be addressed. The minimum number of cells needed to treat the disease needs to be determined. The mouse model is still ideal for these studies.

Scientists envisioned that the first human transplantation would be done with an **autologous transplant,** in which the patient's own bone marrow cells are removed, genetically corrected, and then returned to the patient. In the January 2006 issue of *Nature Biotechnology,* researchers at Sloan-Kettering Cancer Center reported using stem cell-based gene therapy and RNA interference to reverse SCD genetically in human cells. A lentiviral vector carrying a therapeutic globin gene with an embedded small interfering RNA precursor was introduced in the cell cultures of SCD patients to prevent the production of abnormal hemoglobin. The new gene produced normal hemoglobin and suppressed the generation of

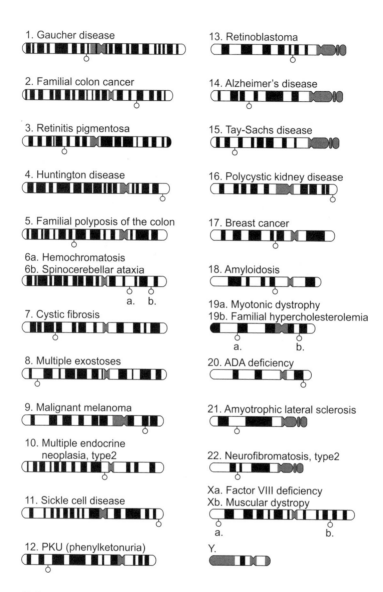

Figure 5-2

Location of single trait genes on chromosomes.

sickle-shaped hemoglobin. Researchers think that this technique can be applied broadly to other malignant cells.

THALASSEMIA: SEA BLOOD

Thalassemia is a group of hereditary anemias occurring in the populations bordering the Mediterranean Sea, in Southeast Asia, and in Africa. The name comes from the Greek *thalassa,* meaning "sea," and *haima,* meaning "blood." This disease affects hemoglobin, the substance in the red blood cells that transports oxygen to the body cells. Normal hemoglobin has a heme molecule and four globins. As in SCD, this condition relates to the types of globins that are produced. A different gene exists for each type of globin, with the exception of alpha-globin, which has two genes.

Humans have genes to construct six types of globins: alpha, beta, gamma, delta, epsilon, and zeta. During embryonic and fetal development, zeta, epsilon, and gamma globins are present, but within weeks after birth, the infant continues to produce alpha-globins, beta-globins, and delta-globins.

In patients with thalassemia, gene mutations in one or more of the globin genes may lead to inadequate levels of related globin. The disease is characterized according to the globin that is affected. The most common types are beta-thalassemia and alpha-thalassemia.

Beta-Thalassemia or Thalassemia Major

When the mutated gene responsible for beta-globin is inherited from both parents, the result is beta-thalassemia major, a severe and life-threatening anemia. During early childhood, the person develops severe anemia, enlargement of the heart and spleen, slight jaundice, and leg ulcers. The younger the child is when the disease occurs, the more unfavorable is the outcome. The condition is also called **Cooley's anemia,** named for the U.S. pediatrician Thomas Cooley (1871–1945), who recognized a condition in which the slightest exertion results in breathlessness and extreme fatigue.

Different symptoms arise according to recessive patterns of inheritance. If only one mutated beta-globin gene is present, symptoms may be few. A person with mild anemia may not be aware that he or she is a carrier. Anemia may appear only during pregnancy or following severe infections. However, inheritance of two mutated genes may cause serious symptoms. Approximately 1 in 150 to 200 children is born with this type; about 2 million Americans carry the trait.

Alpha-Thalassemia or Thalassemia Minor

The alpha-thalassemias are more complex because a person has two alpha-globin genes from each parent, yielding two pairs of genes. If adequate amounts of alpha-globin are produced, the person is a carrier of the trait but has few symptoms. However, if alpha-globin is severely reduced, the offspring may die during fetal development or shortly after birth.

Gene Therapy for Thalassemia

Ryszard Kole and colleagues at the University of North Carolina are investigating the use of a subtle form of gene therapy for thalassemia. As reported by Danny Penman in *New Scientist* (2002), rather than conventional replacement of the gene, the team's approach repairs the dysfunctional messenger RNA (mRNA) that the defective gene produces. By repairing mRNA rather than the damaged gene, the cell's own regulatory mechanisms produce hemoglobin in the correct quantities. Conventional gene therapy approaches often fail because of the control of the proper number of blood cells.

Kole's technique involves getting the hemoglobin-manufacturing system of patients with thalassemia to produce hemoglobin from their own mutated genes. Normal cells transcribe DNA into mRNA, which produces the proteins of hemoglobin. Normal copies of the beta-hemoglobin gene have three coding sites of DNA, interspersed with two non-coding areas, or exons. These non-coding areas are removed in the mRNA. However, short regions bordering the exons indicate the **splice sites,** where the cell cuts and pastes the RNA. In mutations, additional splice sites are added in the mRNA and, when translated, produce malfunctioning hemoglobin molecules.

Using antisense RNA-mirror image sequences of RNA that stick to the additional splice sites, Kole and his team sought to block the additional splice sites. When these sites are blocked, the splicing mechanism can then focus on the original, proper splice sites that produce the normal sequence of mRNA. In this experiment, the bone marrow cells of two patients were genetically modified in vitro to produce antisense RNA. A modified lentivirus inserted the antisense genes into the cell's nuclei. In vitro, the bone marrow cells produced about 20 to 30 percent of a normal person's level of hemoglobin. Kole is in the process of seeking regulatory approval to carry out human trials.

IMMUNE DEFICIENCIES

Without the immune system, hordes of microbes would invade the body, certainly causing death through infection. This all-important system is populated by white blood cells that appear in several forms:

- Granulocytes—cells made of neutrophils, basophils, and eosinophils that have a distinct granular nucleus; these white cells are **phagocytic,** meaning they are able to engulf cells, viruses, and debris.
- Monocytes—cells that consist of one nucleus and that compose the body's first line of defense. Macrophages, the largest member of this group, engulf entire bacteria and damaged or aging cells.
- Lymphocytes—cells that appear to be round and smooth with a large nucleus. The three types are (1) B lymphocytes, which attack foreign matter indirectly by producing antibodies; (2) T lymphocytes, also known as killer T cells, which control and coordinate the immune response by releasing signaling molecules called **cytosines;** they also detect invaders hiding in a cell and can force a cell to "commit suicide" in order to control infection; (3) natural killer (NK) cells.

SCID

SCID, a serious condition that affects the immune system, can be classified according to three types:

- SCID-X1—This disease is carried on the X chromosome. This form results from a mutation in the *IL2RG* gene that causes a receptor for a cytosine called *interleukin-2* to not function (see Chapter 7, X-linked Disorders).

- SCID on chromosome 19—Normally, the IL2R protein activates an important signaling molecule called Janus kinase3 (JAK3). A defect in the *JAK3* gene causes a second type of SCID. In this mutation, defective cytosine receptors and signaling pathways prevent the killer T cells from doing their job.
- ADA located on chromosome 20—The mutation leads to toxic buildup of ADA inside the cells. This condition was the first trial for gene therapy and is profiled in Chapter 4.

Dr. Francesca Santoni de Sio from Milan presented results of a study of children with ADA deficiency at the 2005 American Society of Gene Therapy in St. Louis. Six children had a complete lack of lymphocytes. In the study bone marrow stem cells of the children were harvested and treated with a retroviral vector containing the missing ADA gene. The patients were first treated to reduce production of the mutated cells in the marrow in their bones. They then received a bone marrow transplant with their own marrow that had been corrected by gene therapy. When they came back for follow-up, all six children had cells that were making ADA and able to make lymphocytes. Most of the patients did not require enzyme supplementation of the ADA-PEG drug because the blood-forming cells were making enough ADA to detoxify the rest of the cells. Those who predicted 20 years ago that ADA would be the first condition cured with gene therapy may have been correct.

CYSTIC FIBROSIS: THIEF OF BREATH

Cystic fibrosis (CF), a condition that affects the lungs and pancreas, is one of the most damaging of genetic disorders. Beginning in infancy, the person with CF has thick mucus building up in the respiratory system, is highly susceptible to bacterial infection, and has difficulty breathing. The pancreas malfunctions causing malnutrition. Other organs such as the sweat glands and the liver, do not work properly. In the United States, the disease affects about 1 in 3,900 babies born annually; currently 30,000 Americans are afflicted with this disease. About 1 in 31 Americans—mostly those of Northern European descent—carries the gene. The afflicted person usually dies before the age of 30.

CF is a homozygous recessive disorder, meaning that two copies of the defective allele produce the gene. In 1989 a team of researchers located the gene on the long arm of chromosome 7. One letter causes the mutation in the gene—called the CFTR gene—that codes for the sodium chloride transporter. Normally the transporter is found on the surface of the epithelial cells that line the lungs and other organs, and works like a pump to regulate movement of sodium and chloride in and out of the cells. In people with CF, the pump does not work. Water is retained in the cells, and the tissues do not get the moisture they need. Thus, a dry, sticky mucus builds up in the airways, obstructing breathing, and in the pancreas, interfering with digestion and clogging sweat and salivary glands. Abnormal acid levels build up, making the immune system unable to repel bacteria. A specific bacterium, *Pseudomonas aeruginosa,* is then free to roam and to destroy lung tissue. Traditional treatment involves dislodging the mucus to clear the airways.

Many gene therapy trials for CF are underway. CF is an ideal candidate for gene therapy for the following reasons:

- Scientists know which gene is mutated in the disorder.
- A normal copy of the gene is available.
- The biology of CF is understood, including the types of tissues and how they are affected.
- Scientists can predict that adding the normal gene back to the cells will restore normal function.

The downside of using gene therapy with CF is that animal models are not readily available for testing, and animal modeling is required for preclinical tests. Mice with mutations in the CFTR gene have gastric disturbances only, and do not exhibit the pulmonary effects of CF that occur in humans.

TAY-SACHS DISEASE: PROTECTION AGAINST TUBERCULOSIS

In the late 1880s William Tay (1843–1927), a British ophthalmologist, noted that several Jewish infants with mental and physical retardation had distinct cherry-red spots on the macula and were blind. Later Bernard Sachs (1858–1944), a U.S. neurologist, found a pattern of neurological disturbances in infants with the disease. In addition to physical and mental retardation, the children had an exaggerated startle response, spasticity, convulsions, and enlargement of the head. As the disease progresses, the body loses function, leading to blindness, deafness, paralysis, and death. In the most common forms, the infant begins to show symptoms at about 6 months of age and dies within a few years. A late onset form develops in adolescence and adulthood.

By the late 1940s researchers uncovered the physiological basis of this disease—a deadly accumulation of fatty acids in the brain that destroys nerve cells. By the 1960s investigators discovered that increased levels of an important enzyme caused the accumulation of these toxins in the brain. By the 1970s screenings were conducted for carriers of the defective gene. The disease was named Tay-Sachs after the two physicians who first studied it. In 1989 the defective gene itself was found on chromosome 15. Tay-Sachs disease is a homozygous or single-gene recessive disorder. Two defective alleles—one from each parent—come together to produce the defective gene. According to Mendelian law, if two people who carry the defective gene have a child, the chances are 1 in 4 that the child will have the disorder.

A defect in the HEXA gene, which encodes an enzyme called *hexosaminidase,* causes Tay-Sachs. Hexosaminidase normally breaks down a group of fatty acids called *gangliosides,* but if the HEXA genes do not work properly, gangliosides accumulate in the brain and destroy nerve cells.

Tay-Sachs disease is found especially in the population of Ashkenazi Jews from Eastern Europe. Like several genetic mutations that developed as protection against other conditions, the mutations of Tay-Sachs carriers offer some protection against tuberculosis. Crammed in urban ghettos for many of the past centuries, the

Ashkenazis were especially exposed to the "white death." The protective genes possibly mutated to offer protection at the expense of having lethal effects on some of the population. About 1 in 27 people of Eastern European Jewish descent is thought to be a carrier, and about 1 in 3,600 Jewish infants is born with the disease. The condition is also common among some French-Canadian communities in Quebec and among people from the Cajun country of Louisiana.

Researchers are investigating gene therapy as a cure to the Tay-Sachs disease. Viruses carrying normal cells would be injected to encode enough hexosaminidase to break down accumulating gangliosides. However, a major problem with neurological diseases is getting the payload of large proteins such as genes and enzymes across the blood–brain barrier.

J. E. Guidotti and a French team in 1999 constructed in vitro adenoviral and retroviral vectors to deliver two human subunits of alpha- and beta-hexoaminidases, subunits of the enzyme. Using hex-A-deficient knockout mice, they administered adenoviral vectors coding for both alpha- and beta-subunits. The successful results in mice confirmed that the liver was the preferential target organ to deliver a large amount of secreted proteins.

A 2005 study by Martino et al. combined a nonreplicating *Herpes simplex* virus vector encoding for the hex-A alpha-subunit and a capsule of brain tissue to distribute the missing enzyme. They reestablished the hex-A activity and totally removed the ganglioside buildup in both hemispheres of the brain, in the cerebellum, and in the spinal cord of the Tay-Sachs animal model during 1 month of treatment. In the studies, no adverse effects were observed that were the result of the viral vector, the injection site, or gene expression. However, no human trials on Tay-Sachs are in progress at this time.

GENE THERAPY FOR HEARING

University of Michigan scientists believe that they are one step closer to using gene therapy to grow new auditory hair cells. Reporting in the 1 March 2005 issue of *Nature Medicine*, Yehoash Raphael and associates reported using a pro-hair gene called *Atoh1*, which is normally active only during embryonic development. An adenoviral vector delivered *Atoh1* to the inner ears of adult guinea pigs deafened by ototoxic drugs. Eight weeks later the researchers found new auditory hair cells in the ears treated with *Atoh1*. They tested the animals using brainstem tests, similar to those used to test human hearing. Hearing was better at all frequencies. However, restoration of auditory threshhold levels is not the same as restoring hearing as humans experience it. Therefore, it may be several years before *Atoh1* gene therapy is ready for human testing.

Other single-gene disorders in some stage of research include the following:

- Fanconi anemia—A condition in which the bone marrow fails; also called hypoplastic anemia. A team of researchers at the University of North Carolina, Raleigh, has a phase I clinical trial that transfers corrective gene FAA into progenitor stem cells.
- PNP deficiency—An autosomal recessive disorder of immunity caused by deficiency of an enzyme called *purine nucleoside phosphorylase.*

- PKU—Phenylketonuria, which causes mental retardation if not treated with a special low-phenylalanine diet. PKU may be a good target for gene therapy because the condition affects only one organ and the gene would have to be introduced in only one site.
- Gaucher disease—An inherited condition caused by a mutant gene that inhibits the production of an enzyme called *glucoceregrosidase*. People with the disease have enlarged livers and spleens and their bones eventually deteriorate. Clinical gene therapy focuses on inserting the gene for producing this enzyme.

In a 1984 background paper on gene therapy created by the Office of Technology Assessment, a list was given of diseases for which gene therapy might be considered. At that time researchers foresaw protocols for three types of gene therapy in somatic cells that could be expected in the next few years: immunodeficiency conditions such as ADA or PNP deficiencies; Lesch-Nyhan syndrome; and urea cycle defects such as OTC. Certain metabolic conditions such as Gaucher disease and arginemia were also listed. Expectations for SCD, thalassemias, hemophilias, Tay-Sachs, and CF are not hopeful at all. Those for which gene therapy will probably never be applicable include Down's syndrome, hypertension, and diabetes.

More than 20 years have passed since the publication of this classic document. Dedicated scientists have learned a lot about the genetics of disease. Many researchers have spent a lifetime of research working on just one condition or disorder that they envision can be helped by gene therapy. It is an established principle that diseases caused by single-celled genes should be the simplest to treat. However, scientists are investigating many other genetic disorders caused by single dominant genes, X-linked genes, and multiple gene disorders. Chapters 6, 7, and 8 recount some of the research being done with more complicated inherited patterns.

CHAPTER 6

Single-Gene Traits: Dominant Disorders

George III was the infamous king of Great Britain at the time of the American Revolution. He was also a very ill man. At the age of 50, he experienced abdominal pain and constipation, followed by weak limbs, fever, a fast pulse, and dark red urine. Then nervous system symptoms began, which included insomnia, headaches, restlessness, delirium, convulsions, stupor, and visual problems. His thoughts were confused. He was known to rip off his wig and run about the palace naked while running a high fever. Obviously he was mad. Suddenly the symptoms disappeared, only to return 13 years later and again three years after that. The symptoms always appeared in the same order beginning with the abdominal pain. Finally, in 1811, George went into a prolonged stupor, and the Prince of Wales dethroned him. The doctors of the day were baffled; they had no knowledge that their king had a condition called *porphyria,* an inborn error of metabolism.

In the twentieth century, researchers found the cause of this metabolic condition that makes the urine blood red. The absence of an enzyme causes part of the blood pigment hemoglobin, called the *porphyrin ring,* to be routed into the urine instead of being broken down and metabolized in the cells. Porphyrin then builds up and attacks the nervous system, causing various symptoms. An examination of the pedigree of the British royal family of King George III showed that several relatives had the same symptoms. Porphyria is an example of a single-gene dominant condition.

Dominant disorders occur when a child receives a defective gene from either parent, and the presence of the gene leads to the expression of a genetic defect. In the Mendelian scheme, the trait is dominant.

The figure shows the pattern of dominant inheritance. One affected parent with a dominant mutant gene and a normal recessive, and one unaffected parent with two normal genes have offspring in the following pattern: according to chance, two of the offspring will receive both normal genes and will be normal for the condition, but two of the offspring will receive the dominant gene and will be affected. The likelihood is that 50 percent of the offspring will have the condition

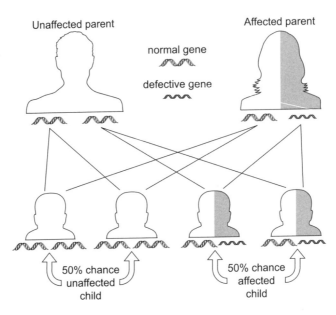

Figure 6-1
Dominant single-gene disorders.

and 50 percent will not. Because the gene is located on an autosomal or body chromosome, both men and women get the disease. Also, the defects occur in people of various ethnic groups.

When diseases are dominant, the gene is powerful and the influence is so strong that the disease develops regardless of efforts to curb it or the influence of the environment. The individual is predestined by the genes to have the disease. Examples of single-gene dominant diseases are Huntington's disease (HD) and porphyria.

HUNTINGTON'S DISEASE: CROWN JEWEL OF GENETIC RESEARCH

On 23 March 1993, Dr. Murray Goldstein, director of the National Institute of Neurological Disorders and Stroke (NINDS), presented the Huntington gene to the world. He said that this gene may prove to be the crown jewel of neurogenetic discoveries. The 10-year search for the gene yielded enormous information about genetic mutations and methods for finding them. The process is considered a model for other genetic research. See the sidebar in this chapter, The Huntington Novel.

According to NINDS, about 30,000 people in the United States have HD— about 1 in 10,000. At least 150,000 people have a 50 percent risk of developing it.

An Old Disease

Early historians documented cases of a strange condition in which normal people in their forties or early fifties began to walk with twitching, jerking, or writhing motions and later began to think and act in bizarre ways. Paracelsus (1492–1541) used the term *chorea,* from the Greek word meaning "dance." This is the same root as in the word *choreography,* in which dancers design their routines. Explanations developed that persons with this bizarre behavior were flirting with the devil. In 1692 Salem residents considered that neighbors exhibiting this dance were possessed by demons and must be burned at the stake.

In 1630 one family from the village of Burres, in Suffolk, England, immigrated to Boston and later descendants moved to Long Island, New York. Several members of this family had chorea. In 1872 Dr. George Huntington of Pomeroy, Ohio, remembered how his father and grandfather, both physicians in New York, cared for this family. He noted that, if either parent had the disease, one or more of the offspring suffered, and described many of the details of the conditions that became known as Huntington's chorea, later as HD. More recently, HD has been called "Woody Guthrie's disease," named for the American folksinger.

HD is an incurable, autosomal, dominant condition resulting from programmed degeneration of the brain cells in an area called the *striatum.* The nerve death is associated with uncontrolled movements, loss of intellectual faculties, and emotional disturbance. Most of those affected develop HD in the middle of adult life. However, 10 percent have an early-onset form, beginning before the age of 20 and called juvenile HD; and another 10 percent show symptoms of HD after age 55. Because HD is on an autosomal gene, men and women inherit the gene equally. The disease affects all ethnic groups but is more common among those of European descent. Patients may live 10 to 15 years after the start of the symptoms.

Each child of a parent with the disease has a 50–50 chance of inheriting the gene, which is associated with a repeat of the cytosine-adenine-guanine (CAG) triplet repeats located on chromosome 4p 16.3; the gene is named *huntingtin.*

The discovery in 1993 resulted in a genetic test for diagnosis. The test analyzes DNA by counting the number of CAG repeats. Those people who have 28 or fewer repeats do not have HD. A number of people have borderline repeats and may pass the condition on to successive generations. If a person has 40 or more repeats, that individual will develop HD, as shown in Table 6-1.

Finding a gene and finding a cure are very different things. One scientist has stated that so many people are doing research on HD that finding enough people to study is becoming a problem. Understanding the basic biology is still very important. Unraveling the mechanism of HD shows that patients with the disease produce cells in which an abnormal protein breaks into smaller, toxic pieces that clog the cells. The toxic fragments appear to impair the mitochondria and get into the nucleus of the cells, causing the wrong genes to be put into action.

Genetic Therapy Trials

University of British Columbia researchers have cured HD in a mouse model. An article by Emily Chung (2006) cites the explanation given by Michael Hayden, director of the Centre for Molecular Medicine and Therapeutics, of how researchers found an abnormal protein (also called huntingtin) that breaks into fragments that are toxic to the brain. By stopping the action of an enzyme called *caspase-6,* which degrades the huntingtin protein into fragments, researchers

Table 6-1   HD Outcome According to CAG Repeats

Number of CAG Repeats	Outcomes
Less than or equal to 28	Normal range. The individual will not develop HD.
29–34	The individual will not develop HD, but the next generation is at risk.
35–39	Some but not all individuals will develop HD; the next generation is at risk.
Greater than or equal to 40	The individual will develop HD; it will pass to the next generation at a ratio of 50:50.

Source: Evelyn B. Kelly, adapted from http://www.ninds.nih.gov.

prevented disease symptoms in genetically engineered mice. When the animals were sacrificed, their brains appeared normal. Hayden said that the groups will continue their work on genetic alterations to block the enzymes, as well as add drugs to block the enzyme.

Gene therapy has been suggested as a way to switch off genes to slow down HD. The method, called **RNA interference,** involves a natural defense mechanism against viruses. In this process, short pieces of double-stranded RNA, called *short interfering RNAs (siRNAs),* trigger the degrading of other RNA in the cell with a matching sequence. If a siRNA is chosen to match the RNA copied from a particular gene, it will stop the production of the protein that the gene codes for. Applying this knowledge to HD, researchers know that mutation in the *huntingtin* gene results in the defective protein causing large clumps that gradually kill part of the brain cells.

Beverly Davidson at the University of Iowa found that reducing production of the defective protein slows down the disease (Holmes, 2002). Even reducing levels of the toxic protein by a small amount can have an impact. In 2002 Davidson's team found that, by adding DNA that codes for siRNA to rodent cells engineered to produce the protein, the amount of a similar protein is reduced. The team was the first to use gene therapy to deliver the huntingtin protein. One of the problems with *huntingtin* is that completely silencing the gene in people is not an option because brain cells may not survive without the protein. But people with HD have two copies of the gene, and only one is defective. Other researchers have shown that siRNA can recognize and silence only the mutant gene. Davidson and her team found that a change in a single DNA letter appears in 70 percent of the defective genes. Adding siRNA that matches the sequence reduced the expression of the defective protein by 80 percent without affecting the normal protein. Research into siRNA is still in its infancy, but investigators envision this technique as a possible tool for curing many genetic disorders.

FAMILIAL HYPERCHOLESTEROLEMIA (FHC)

FHC is caused by a defective gene on chromosome 19 that codes for an abnormal receptor protein unable to mediate the uptake of cholesterol into cells. As a result, cholesterol builds up in the blood and may eventually lead to **arterioscle-rosis** or **coronary** heart disease. FHC is an autosomal dominant disorder in which the presence of only one abnormal allele in one parent is necessary for the offspring to have the disease.

AMYOTROPHIC LATERAL SCLEROSIS (ALS): LOU GEHRIG'S DISEASE

During the Babe Ruth glory years for the New York Yankees, a player named Lou Gehrig became the favorite of the fans. However, after several years the coaches and fans recognized that Gehrig was struggling in playing the game. He revealed to the team and fans that he had a fatal disease that would eventually cause him to lose all control of movement. The disease, amyotrophic lateral sclerosis (ALS), was called "Lou Gehrig's disease" after the popular player.

ALS is a neurological condition in which all motor neurons express a high level of the mutant gene *mutant SOD1*. However, researchers have developed an antisense oligonucleotide, delivered through the spine, that in mouse models silences the gene coding for the protein.

POLYCYSTIC KIDNEY DISEASE

This inherited disease causes the kidneys to develop fluid-filled cavities or cysts that are major causes of kidney failure in children and adults. The most common condition is autosomal dominant polycystic kidney disease (ADPKD). There is also a recessive type that causes kidney disease in children. ADPKD affects 60,000 persons in the United States and 12.5 million worldwide.

Researchers have found that a chemical compound known as cyclic AMP is largely responsible for the cell buildup and fluid secretion that cause the kidney cysts to develop. Inhibition of the chemicals that cause this buildup is a target for gene therapy.

NEUROFIBROMATOSES (NF)

NF is actually a group of diseases with common symptoms caused by mutations in the DNA of two different genes. The common elements include neurofibromas—soft, noncancerous tumors—from the nerves and café-au-lait-colored spots. There are two types of NF:

- NF1—This type involves a mutation in the *NF1* gene that makes the protein neurofibromin. When this protein does not work properly, growth is not under control and tumors form on the nerves. Because this is an autosomal dominant condition, the patient with type 1 NF has a 50 percent chance of passing the gene to his or her offspring regardless of gender. There is a mouse model of *NF1* and gene therapy is a possibility.
- NF2—This type is much less common and involves a different gene. It is caused by a mutation in the DNA of a gene called *NF2*, which makes the

protein merlin. People with NF2 are likely to get tumors of the nerve for hearing and balance called *vestibular schwannomas,* which may cause deafness and loss of balance.

FAMILIAL HYPERTROPHIC CARDIOMYOPATHY: MARFAN SYNDROME

Several autosomal dominant conditions are very complex, and scientists face considerable difficulty in understanding the biological paths of the diseases, which are necessary for gene therapy. The typical scenario is the following: A healthy young teenager dies of sudden heart failure, and the autopsy shows the cause of death to be an inherited heart disorder. The boy's father had died at a young age, as had the paternal grandmother and paternal great-uncle. This autosomal dominant condition does not skip generations, and it affects both sexes.

Dominant disorders can be problematic because the condition does not appear until the person is past childbearing age. For example, most people with HD develop it after their children are born. Also, many die suddenly as young adults, as in Marfan syndrome. Dominant disorders are not as prevalent as recessive disorders. Also, in most of these dominant disorders, the biochemical nature of the derangement of the mutation is just being developed. An autosomal dominant trait does not skip generations, and it can affect both sexes. Transmission stops when an individual does not inherit the causative gene. The molecular defects in dominant disorders have proven to be much more difficult, but new techniques under development, especially in siRNA, may ultimately be effective for treating these disorders.

The Huntington Novel

The story of the discovery of the Huntington gene reads almost like a novel. Southern novelist William Faulkner was interested in family diseases and charted large families with unique disorders for his stories of fictional Mississippi towns. Whereas Faulkner used keen writing skill to produce literary masterpieces, geneticists use scientific data to chart large families in real situations.

Nancy Wexler, a New York psychologist, saw her mother die of HD and realized that she had a 50–50 chance of inheriting her mother's disease. Watching a film on the Discovery Channel, she saw villagers on Lake Maracaibo in Venezuela walking with the writhing dance reminiscent of Huntington's chorea. In 1978 she received a grant to go to the village, where she convinced people to donate blood samples. She charted the family tree of the villagers, showing the presence or absence of the trait in

---

10,000 people. The gene was traced to a Portuguese sailor who had introduced the mutant gene in the nineteenth century. Wexler provided 2,000 blood samples to the Harvard research team of molecular biologist James Gusella. They expected it would take years to find a marker that traveled with the gene, but amazingly, on the third try they found DNA patterns from healthy relatives to be distinct from those with HD. Thus, researchers were able to trace the gene to the tip of the short arm of chromosome 4.

CHAPTER 7

X-Linked Disorders

When the famous chemist John Dalton (1766–1844) and his brother looked at the world, they saw it differently than other people. When they looked at sealing wax that appeared red to most individuals, they saw it as green, like a leaf. Pink wildflowers were blue. Dalton was very curious about this strange phenomenon, and he willed his eyeballs to medical science in the hope that researchers, after his death, would one day find the reason for his colorblindness. Later geneticists realized that his colorblind condition was a sex-linked recessive trait carried on the X chromosome. In the United States 7 percent of males and 0.4 percent of females are colorblind.

When a gene is passed on only the X chromosome, it is a sex-linked gene. As chromosomes go, the X chromosome is large and may be considered odd or a misfit. Its mate in a pair, the Y chromosome, is a tiny, almost inert stub. The X and Y chromosomes, or sex chromosomes, determine sex. Everybody gets an X from his or her mother, but inheriting an X from the father creates a female; if one inherits a Y, the individual becomes a male.

The term *X-linked trait* refers to traits found on the X chromosome. X-linked traits such as John Dalton's colorblindness are more frequent in males, who have only one X chromosome.

Some X-linked traits are merely annoying, and people with the trait manage to adapt to its conditions. Some traits are cosmetically undesirable. For example, a middle-aged man had a terrible skin condition called *ichthyosis,* in which his skin looked scaly like a fish. He realized it was an inherited trait when his daughter's son showed the same condition. Many other sex-linked traits are serious and life-threatening (see list in Table 7-1).

Although inherited disorders such as colorblindness and ichthyosis are annoying, these cosmetically undesirable conditions are not candidates for gene therapy. However, several life-threatening X-linked traits have been the target of gene therapy studies. Unfortunately, drugs and other treatments for conditions such as SCID-X and hemophilia are very expensive—and they are not working.

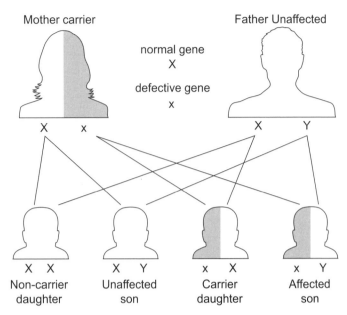

Figure 7-1
Pattern of X-linked inheritance.

Gene therapists hope to provide a more permanent cure for many of these lethal conditions.

X-LINKED SCID: IMMUNE DEFICIENCY

People go through life taking their immune systems for granted. However, without an immune system, all animals would face death from a multitude of diseases. The immune system is rich in white blood cells, or leucocytes, that have several forms: T cells, B cells, and microphages. Here are their functions:

- T cells control the immune response as they release signaling molecules called *cytosines* that call on B cells and microphages. T cells may also detect invaders hiding in a cell and may even force them to "commit suicide."
- B cells produce antibodies that attack invading bodies.
- Microphages confront the invaders head-on by eating them. They are called phagocytic cells.

But what happens when one of the genes that control the action of the signaling bodies is faulty? No action can occur. This is what happens in the several forms of SCID.

SCID-X1, called X-linked SCID, is a disease that destroys the immune system and is fatal unless precautions are taken. Located on the X chromosome, the faulty gene is passed on by the mother to sons. The gene that makes the immune protein interleukin-2, or the *IL2RG* gene, causes SCID-X. This *IL2RG* gene activates a molecule—JAK3, an important signaling molecule. However, if the defective gene is present, cytosine receptors and blocked signaling molecules prevent normal development of the T lymphocytes. The male infant is born with a compromised immune system that makes him susceptible to any diseases in his environment. Sometimes, the boy can be kept alive (although not for long) in a bubble or large plastic encasement that keeps him away from microorganisms.

In 2000 Alan Fischer at Necker Hospital in Paris carried out the first gene therapy treatment for X-SCID. This successful trial was proclaimed a great breakthrough. A handful of other trials were performed in Great Britain. In April 2002 the mother of a Welsh boy who had been treated at Great Ormond Street hospital described her son's progress as "nothing short of a miracle." Pleased with the possibilities, scientists had treated a total of 15 patients: 11 in Paris and 4 in London.

However, the so-called miracle was short-lived. In October 2002 one of the boys developed leukemia as a direct consequence of the treatment. The boy had undergone gene therapy at the age of 6 months, but at the age of two and a half he contracted chickenpox. His white blood cells increased in response to the infection (which would not have occurred without the treatment), but then the marrow started uncontrollably producing white blood cells. While the government investigated, the boy underwent chemotherapy for his leukemia and progressed well.

The scientists explained that, because the genes were put into the boy's cells using a harmless virus, the doctors could not target the gene to a specific part of a chromosome. In this boy, the new gene was inserted next to an oncogene called *Lmo2,* thus triggering leukemia.

In France the gene therapy trials were halted, but the Gene Therapy Advisory Committee (GTAC) in Great Britain recognized that although unanticipated, this type of side effect was always possible. The GTAC confirmed that all protocols had been followed. Although some children are candidates for bone marrow transplant treatments, others die without gene therapy. The GTAC confirmed that gene therapy treatments would continue in the United Kingdom. Two UK boys died while awaiting the decision to continue therapy.

Mark Bodine, Senior Investigator at the National Human Genome Research Institute, said that although the adverse events were a shock because at one point everything was going so well, it is important to note that the group included all 13 patients being treated. Of the 13 children, in one patient the graft did not "take," and in another the gene transfer was very poor. Of the remaining 11 patients, 3 experienced adverse events, but 2 of these 3 patients responded immediately to therapy and now have a fully functional immune system. So 11 of the 13 were treated, and 10 of these children are now alive. With conventional treatments, this number would be much lower. See Chapter 14 for the suggestions of scientists Fischer and Cavazzana-Calvo on how to improve treatments.

HEMOPHILIA

Hemophilia has a noble place in history although the disease itself is a killer. In 1828 the German physician Johann Schonlein (1793–1864) used the term

Table 7-1 Conditions Caused by Disease-Related Genes on the Human X Chromosome

Eye Conditions	Inborn Errors of Metabolism	Nerve and Muscle Conditions	Other Conditions
Green colorblindness, abnormal green cones in the retina	Agammaglobulinemia, lack of certain antibodies	Charcott-Marie-Tooth Disease, loss of feeling in the ends of the arms and legs	Amelogenesis imperfecta, abnormal tooth enamel
Megalocornea (enlarged cornea)	Granulomatous disease, skin and lung infections, enlarged liver and spleen	Fragile X-syndrome, mental retardation, enlarged face and testicles	Alport syndrome, deafness, inflamed kidneys
Norrie disease, abnormal growth of the retina	Diabetes insipidus, frequent urination	Hydrocephalus (excess fluid on the brain)	Cleft palate, opening in the roof of the mouth
Ocular albinism (no eye pigment)	Fabry disease, abdominal pains, kidney failure	Lesch-Nyhan syndrome, mental retardation	Hypohidrotic ectodermal dysplasia; absence of teeth, hair, and sweat glands
Red colorblindness	Gout, inflamed joints	Menkes disease, kinky hair, abnormal copper transport	Ichthyosis (rough scaly skin)
Retinitis pigmentosa, clumps of pigment in the eye	G6PD deficiency and favism, anemia after eating fava beans	Becker and Duchenne muscular dystrophy, progressive muscle weakness	Incontinentia pigmenti, skin color marked with swirls like marbled cake
Retinoschisis, the retina degenerates and splits	Hemophilia A and B, blood does not clot	Spinal and bulbar muscular atrophy, muscle weakness	Kallman syndrome, the inability to smell; undeveloped testes

Hypophosphatemia, rickets

Testicular feminization (the male embryo does not respond to male hormones; appears female)

Hunter syndrome, deformed face, dwarfism

Ornithine transcarbamylase deficiency, ammonia accumulation in the blood

Primary adrenal hypoplasia, affects the adrenal glands

SCID, lack of immune cells

Wiskott-Aldrich syndrome, too few blood platelets

Created by Evelyn B. Kelly.

hemophiliac to describe a group of patients who were predisposed to bleeding and hemorrhaging. In history, the Jewish Talmud referred to a bleeding disorder and excused from circumcision the boys whose mother had lost several sons to this disorder. In the tenth century, Islamic surgeon Abu al-Qasim also described a bleeding disorder. More recently, the fates of several royal families of Europe traced a recessive mutation that occurred on the X chromosome of Queen Victoria of England. Through intermarriage, the condition spread to the courts of Russia, Germany, and Spain. Accounts describe the young Russian prince Alexander, a victim of hemophilia, wailing in pain throughout the massive palace in St. Petersburg.

A simple paper cut on the finger calls up a process of blood clotting that involves a complex process of enzymes and protein factors. For example, two clotting factors—VIII and IX—activate a third factor, XI, to stimulate the proteins prothrombin, thrombin, and fibrinogen to produce fibrin, the substance of the clot. In hemophilia the clotting factors are partly or completely missing. Hemophilia is classified according to these three types:

- Hemophilia A, caused by the absence of clotting protein factor VIII
- Hemophilia B, caused by the absence of clotting protein factor IX
- Hemophilia C, caused by the absence of clotting protein factor XI

These three factors are essential to the formation of the clot of fibrin.

Hemophilia is a classic example of X-chromosomal recessive inheritance in humans. If males receive the defective gene from their mothers, they will have the condition because no normal gene is present on the X chromosome. Females have such genes compensated for by a normal gene, but they will be carriers of the mutant allele. A male hemophiliac generally has healthy offspring—although the daughters are carriers; none of his sons possess the gene. The condition is rare in females because they must inherit both genes from parent carriers. On the average, 1 in 5,000 males has hemophilia A, and 1 in 25,000 has hemophilia B.

For many years, blood transfusions were the conventional treatment for hemophilia, but repeated injections led to liver damage and, in recent times, to contamination of the blood supply by HIV. In the 1980s many hemophiliacs developed AIDS from the transfusion procedure. In the early 1990s genetically engineered blood factors were developed. The normal gene is cloned into cell lines that can produce large amounts of human factor VIII.

Gene therapy would directly replace the faulty gene in the patient. According to logic, treating hemophilia should be the gold standard in gene therapy. Hemophilia is a single-gene disease for which the gene was cloned several years ago. Generating a lot of protein is not necessary; only 5 percent of normal levels is sufficient to prevent or shorten bleeding episodes. It is easy to tell whether the therapy is working by measuring the factor VIII or IX and testing for clotting. The market is there. For the 17,000 people with hemophilia, the cost of treatment with recombinant factor VIII or IX costs $1,000 or more per treatment (about $100,000 annually). Although gene therapy may not be cheaper at first, it would open a competitive market that would eventually lead to lower treatment prices.

At least seven biotechnology companies have entered the race to develop gene therapy for hemophilia (see list in Table 7-2).

Table 7-2 Biotechnology Firms in the Race for Hemophilia Gene Therapy

Company	Vector or Delivery	Status
Chiron Corp., Emeryville, CA	Retrovirus	Phase I
Avigen Inc., Alameda, CA	Adeno-associated virus	Phase I
Transkaryotic Therapies, Inc., Cambridge, MA	Ex vivo transfection	Phase I
GTI/SysStemix (a division of Novartis) Gaitherburg, MD and Palo Alto, CA	Adenovirus	Preclinical
Cell Genesis, Inc., Foster City, CA	Adeno-associated virus	Preclinical
Kimeragen, Inc., Newtown, PA	Chimeric oligonucleotides	Preclinical
GenStar, San Diego, CA	Several strategies	Preclinical

Created by Evelyn B. Kelly.

Chiron, the oldest company in competition, has used the retrovirus vectors to deliver treatment to hemophiliac rabbits and dogs in a phase I safety study. Chiron investigators have found that the liver is an ideal place for gene targeting, but have yet to resolve one question related to the amounts of gene necessary for humans, who have much more body mass than dogs or rabbits. Another company, GTI, is betting on adenoviruses to deliver the payload. However, when the AD viruses went into mice (and eventually into humans) for safety testing, gene expression sputtered and crashed. Improving the virus by moving certain backbone genes may still be an answer. Avigen Inc. is inserting adeno-associated viruses into the thigh muscles of patients with hemophilia B.

As of 2006 tests were still in preclinical or phase I safety status. Will any of these experimental treatments cure hemophilia? Time will tell.

DUCHENNE MUSCULAR DYSTROPHY

In the nineteenth century Guillaume Duchenne (1805–1875), a French neurologist, described a condition usually occurring in childhood, in which mostly boys developed a clumsy, waddling gait and had difficulty getting up from the floor. The condition named for this doctor became known as Duchenne muscular dystrophy (DMD). It is one of a group of dystrophinopathies that show a progressive degeneration of the skeletal muscles. DMD occurs at a frequency of 1 per 3,500 live births. Around ages 9 to 12, the child loses the ability to walk. As people with DMD get older, the pace of muscle fiber loss increases, and they usually die in their third decade.

DMD is caused by an X-linked recessive abnormal gene, and occurs more frequently among males than females. The pattern of inheritance follows the general scheme for X-linked conditions. Males need only one mutant gene to have the disease because they have only one X chromosome; females do not express the condition unless the gene is on both X chromosomes.

The hereditary disease is caused by a mutation in the DMD gene that is located on chromosome X. The gene codes for a protein dystrophin, which strengthens muscle cells as it anchors the cytoskeleton to the surface membrane. Without dystrophin, the muscle's cell membrane lets fluid enter, which causes it to swell and rupture from high internal pressure.

Some patients have severe muscular dystrophy for one of two reasons:

- They have complete deletion of the gene.
- They have a **stop codon** that shortens the gene. For these patients, suppressing the stop codon might allow the cell to make the normal protein.

The mouse knockout model of DMD helps researchers understand the role of dystrophin in muscle physiology. Researchers conducting gene therapy trials in mice are attempting to replace the mutated dystrophin or to introduce a closely related substance, utrophin, to stabilize the cell's membranes. Because the gene is so large, it would be difficult to put it into a cell, so other gene therapy techniques must be used.

Aurelie Goyenvalle and her colleagues (2005) found that DNA has multiple coding sequences interspersed with noncoding introns that are spliced out during RNA processing. The gene therapy vector delivers a specially engineered gene called *U7,* which is transcribed into an RNA molecule that perfectly matches the DNA segment containing a stop codon. The bad sequence that has the stop codon is looped out and continues to make the proper protein. Mice that have been treated with the process are walking fine. The problem is that humans have much larger muscles than mice. Possibly targeting a smaller muscle area, such as the diaphragm or the hands, could make a difference.

RETINITIS PIGMENTOSA (RP)

Some conditions may be transmitted by many genes that cause the mutation. Retinitis pigmentosa (RP) is one of the conditions that have been traced to more than 100 different genes. RP is a group of inherited eye diseases that affect the retina or light-sensitive part of the eye. RP causes the breakdown of photoreceptor cells in the retina that detect light. As these cells break down and die, patients experience progressive vision loss.

The gene may be autosomal recessive, autosomal dominant, or X-linked recessive. Sex-linked RP has been traced to a specific area of the X chromosome, and has been mentioned as a candidate for gene therapy. However, there are currently no trials on RP at the National Human Genome Research Institute (NHGRI).

X-LINKED RETINOSCHISIS

Researchers at the University of Florida used a healthy human gene to prevent blindness in mice that had a form of an incurable eye disease that strikes boys. Retinoschisis is first detected in boys between 5 and 10 years of age, when their vision problems cause reading difficulties. In a healthy eye, retinal cells secrete a protein called *retinoschisin* (RSI), which acts like a glue to connect the layers of the retina. Without it, the retinal layers separate and tiny cysts form, often leading to blindness.

The University of Florida researchers injected a healthy version of the human *RSI* gene into the subretinal space of the right eyes of genetically engineered 15-day-old mice. Six months later, using a laser ophthalmoscope, the doctors found cysts in the untreated eyes, but the treated eyes appeared healthy. The protein in the retina indicated that the changes were long-lasting, an encouraging sign that the treatment may be able to repair retinal damage. Researchers are planning to submit requests for phase I trials in human patients. The procedure may prove effective for not only retinoschisis, but also for other conditions of the eye, such as RP.

X-LINKED CHRONIC GRANULOMATOUS DISEASE

In April 2006 researchers reported in *Nature Medicine* that gene therapy had been used for the first time to correct a myeloid immunodeficiency. Myelocytes are large cells in the bone marrow from which white blood cells are derived. Chronic granulomatous disease is an immunodeficiency caused by a mutation in the gene *gp91phox,* which leads to phagocytes with impaired ability to fight microbes. Dr. Christof von Kalle from the National Center for Tumor Diseases in Heidelberg, Germany, and his colleagues treated two patients with gene therapy and found a large number of functioning phagocytes. According to the authors, gene transfer into hematopoietic stem cells has been successful in correcting lymphoid immunodeficiencies, but not myeloid ones.

ORNITHINE TRANSCARBAMYLASE (OTC) DEFICIENCY

OTC, which received so much publicity from a failed gene therapy experiment in 1999, is an X-linked metabolic condition in which the body cannot get rid of ammonia. Half of the children with OTC die within their first month of life; others die before their fifth birthday. Jesse Gelsinger had a mild form of the disease; some of his enzymes were functioning normally. (The story of this ill-fated experiment is in Chapter 11. Also see Appendix A for details of the lawsuit against the University of Pennsylvania.)

Many other X-linked genes are candidates for gene therapy, including the following:

- Adrenoleukodystrophy—A recessive sex-linked trait that causes abnormality of the white matter of the brain and atrophy of the adrenal glands, leading to mental and physical deterioration; there is no cure.
- Lesch-Nyhan syndrome—A condition occurring only in males, in which children are mentally retarded, become extremely aggressive, and often mutilate themselves by biting their own lips or fingers. Patients with this disease do not manufacture the **hypoxanthine guanine** phosphoribosyl-transferase enzyme. The normal version of the gene has been cloned. Unfortunately, mouse models have only mild symptoms of Lesch-Nyhan because there is an alternative metabolic pathway. The different pathway renders the mouse not suitable for use as a model.

CHAPTER 8

Multigene and Traits Influenced by the Environment

The fat little fur ball is huddled in the corner of his cage after hours of eating. His name O.B., which stands for obesity, fits him perfectly—his only desires in life appear to be eating and sleeping. Born in 1950 at Jackson Laboratory in Bar Harbor, Maine, O.B. and other mutants became serious subjects in the study of the genetics of obesity.

At first glance, the problem of obesity, which has been proclaimed a world epidemic, is considered simple: eat too much, gain weight; exercise and diet, lose weight. However, a few single-gene conditions, such as Berardinelli syndrome and Prader-Willi syndrome, are characterized by morbid obesity that is not simple. For most people, the problem is a complex combination of genes, food intake, inadequate activity, environment, and family traditions. Genes may even control some environmental choices, such as appetite and overeating. Sensational stories are often in the news about the elusive "fat gene," "couch potato gene," "stop eating gene," "can't resist gene," and even a "party platter gene." The study of the genetics of obesity is snowballing, and genes that affect obesity have been identified (see list in Table 8-1).

Obesity is a prime example of multigenes interacting with the environment. Ongoing studies are at the basic level; the few that have reached the clinical level usually include drug intervention. Obesity researchers are hoping that people will someday benefit from gene therapy. Two researchers at the University of Florida used gene therapy to stimulate the brain protein proopiomelanocortin (POMC) in obese, diabetic mice and found that this system may be affected by age-related obesity. Future gene therapy may be able to target some of these genes. A problem with social issues such as obesity is that some people want to undergo these procedures for cosmetic purposes. As emphasized in Chapters 9, 10, 11, and 12,

Table 8-1   Selected Genes and Their Influence on Obesity

Gene	Mechanism	Gene Effect
Leptins (OB or LEP)	Appetite, energy expenditure	Major
Leptin receptors (OB-R or LEP-R)	Appetite, energy expenditure	Major
Uncoupling protein-1 (UCP-1)	Energy expenditure	Minor
Uncoupling protein-2 (UCP-2)	Raised body temperature, requiring increased calories	Minor
Proopiomelanocortin (POMC)	Appetite	Major
Melanocortin-4 receptor (MC4-R)	Appetite	Major
Peroxisome proliferator-activated receptors (PPAR-γ-1 and -2)	Adipocyte differentiation; insulin	Major

Adapted from Evelyn Kelly's *Obesity*, Greenwood Press, 2006.

ethicists and regulatory bodies agree that gene therapy for cosmetic enhancement is not appropriate.

Multigene traits are those caused by several genes. Many characteristics, such as eye or hair color, do not follow simple inheritance or Mendelian patterns. These disorders are referred to as *polygenic* or *multigenic*. Other traits may be present in the genes, but they do not appear unless the behavior or environment is present to modify the trait. These environmentally modified traits, which combine genetic predisposition and interaction with the environment, determine the vast majority of characteristics. For example, height is influenced by nutrition and other factors. Many diseases derive from the interaction of genes with the environment.

These multigenic conditions generally do not appear to be the best targets for gene therapy, but some successes have been indicated. This chapter considers some of the research using gene therapy for cancer, neurological diseases, cardiovascular diseases, diabetes, musculoskeletal conditions, HIV, problems of surgery, and macular degeneration.

GENE THERAPY AND CANCER

Hippocrates noted in 400 BC that the veins radiating from a breast cancer resembled the legs of a crab and gave it the name *karkinoma* in Greek, which became *cancer* in Latin. In 1775 Percival Potts, a London doctor, found the first clues to the cause when he noted that chimney sweeps had a high incidence of scrotal cancer. Later it was found that radiation caused cancer: Marie Curie, the discoverer of X-rays, died of malignant skin cancer.

Actually, cancer is not a single disease, but many different diseases that share common biological characteristics. The disease may develop in any tissue and at any age. Cancer is a genetic disease at the cellular level. The hallmark of a malignant cancer is the uncontrolled spread of abnormal cancer cells. Cancer is the most common genetic disease, but only rarely is it directly inherited. Most cancers are sporadic and arise in certain tissues, such as the colon, breast, lung, or skin. Cancers arise through a multistage process driven by inherited and relatively frequent somatic mutations of cellular genes, followed by cloning of the abnormal cells that grow aggressively.

Three important classes of related genes are targeted by mutations:

- Protooncogenes
- Tumor suppressor genes
- DNA repair genes

In some young people with cancers, germ-line mutations of tumor suppressor, or DNA repair, genes are the primary cause. However, in contrast to germ-line gene therapy approaches, somatic gene therapy approaches are not suitable for treating patients harboring a germ-line mutation for the cancer-causing gene. In these individuals, all cells—at least in some tissues—are at risk for cancer development.

However, the vast majority of mutations that contribute to cancer are somatic. Treatment possibilities include introduction of a gene that might alter or inhibit the malignant phenotype into the cancer cells.

Because there are many different kinds of cancer, several different types of gene therapy are employed in targeting cancer. The most common diseases include breast and ovarian cancer, colon cancer, and melanoma.

Breast and Ovarian Cancer

Breast cancer involves the changing of one or more genes. Although viruses may have a role in some cancers, the mechanism still involves changing genetic material that is similar to that of a natural mutation. Breast cancer is the leading cause of death in women between the ages of 30 and 50 and is second only to heart disease as a cause of death in women over 50. Approximately 1 woman in 10 develops breast cancer in her lifetime. Also, about 1,000 men develop this cancer each year.

Although the vast majority of breast and ovarian cancers are sporadic forms of the disease, about 5 to 10 percent of malignancy cases are hereditary or familial. Of the hereditary cases, mutations in the *BRCA1* or *BRCA2* genes are currently associated with 30 to 70 percent of all breast cancer cases and 90 percent of ovarian cancer cases. Possible mutations in other genes are currently under investigation.

BRCA1 and *BRCA2* are located on autosomes. The mutated genes appear to be dominant, making the chance of passing the mutated gene to progeny 50 percent. Women with the mutant genes have risk rates varying from 16 percent for women under age 30, to 63 percent or more for women over the age of 55. These genes almost always cause the disease in a given family. However, a second mutation from the other parent is required for the malignancy to occur.

BRCA1 and *BRCA2* belong to a class of genes known as *tumor suppressor genes,* which control cell growth. Normally, these suppressor genes keep cells within their normal tissue boundaries and play an important role in signaling the cell pathways that control cell death when damage is detected. Mutations of the tumor suppressor genes decrease the control capabilities.

BRCA1 is composed of 5,500 base pairs located on chromosome 17. A base pair is A/T, T/A, G/C, or C/G. Every sequence of three base pairs is a codon that encodes for a specific polypeptide, known as an *amino acid.* Mutations can occur at any place in the gene structure and can thus program for a variety of proteins, depending on the place of the change. The mutated gene products, called *onco-proteins,* cannot play a normal role in the cell's development. These foreign proteins may then trigger mechanisms that interfere with other genes and inhibit the cellular levels of neighboring proteins. Oncoproteins can lead to breast cancer, ovarian cancer, benign forms of overgrowth, and structural damage to the paired allele. Uncontrolled growth leads to cancer or tumors, invasion of neighboring tissue, and later to mass migration of malignant cells (i.e., metastasis) through the lymphatic system, blood, or to distant organs such as the brain, bones, and liver.

BRCA2 was the second gene to be discovered. In 1994 scientists studying Icelandic families found a perfect genetic laboratory: a population that had immigrated from Norway in 900 AD and become isolated, with little influx into its genetic pool. Virtually all of the 270,000 Icelanders trace their ancestry to the few thousand Vikings who came to the island and inbred. The incidence of breast cancer is high in this population. The gene, located on chromosome 13, consists of about 11,000 base pairs. In addition to cancer in female members of the population, male members also tend to develop breast cancer or prostate cancer.

Several gene therapy trials are attempting to replace or supplement the mutated genes with normal copies. Some trials are also seeking to put tumor suppressor genes into breast cells to block development of cancer growth.

Malignant Melanoma

Melanoma is an aggressive, malignant form of skin cancer characterized by irregular black moles. Every year more than 40,000 people in North America are diagnosed with melanoma, and about 8,500 individuals die from the condition. Overexposure to the harmful radiation of the sun causes melanoma, which often reoccurs although treatment may cause remission.

Melanoma has been traced to a mutation in a gene on chromosome 9, known as cyclin-dependent kinase N2, or *CDKN2*. The gene makes the person susceptible to this form of cancer. *CDKN2* codes for protein p16, which regulates cell division and the timing of DNA synthesis. When protein p16 is defective, uncontrolled cell division occurs.

In August 2006 scientists at the U.S. National Cancer Institute (NCI) announced in the journal *Science* the success of gene therapy in two patients with advanced melanoma. The two patients were among a cohort of 17 patients, 15 of whom did not respond to the treatment. The patients were both males in the last stages of the illness. The 53-year-old patient, whose cancer had metastasized to the liver and lymph glands, had a complete regression in the axilla mass and an

89-percent reduction in the liver mass, which was then removed surgically. The 30-year-old patient had developed a mass in the lung, but after treatment the cancer regressed. Both were clinically free of cancer about 19 months after treatment.

The new technique, as reported by Stephen Rosenberg, involves taking normal lymphocytes and infecting them with a retrovirus encoding a T-cell-receptor (TCR) gene. The gene activates the lymphocytes into tumor recognition. The researchers used genes encoding TCR specific for melanoma antigen (MART-1).

However, the scientists were excited about the technique of manipulating normal lymphocytes taken from the patients, which represents the first time that gene therapy has been used successfully to treat cancer. They are hoping that the procedure will be applicable to a broad range of common cancers.

RNA Interference for Cancer Therapy

RNA interference (RNAi) is a powerful gene-silencing process that holds great promise in the field of cancer therapy. RNAi regulates the expression of genes, which determines cell fate and differentiation. Considerable progress has been made in understanding how RNAi mediates gene silencing. Understanding the molecular pathways that are important for carcinogenesis has created the opportunity to use RNAi technology to target key molecules in the pathway.

High-throughput technology, a sophisticated process that enables the study of many substances at one time, has enhanced the profiling of cancer cells and of the genes that are dysregulated in cancers. B. Vogelstein and K. W. Kinzler (2004) have listed the major cellular pathways altered in cancer:

- The receptor protein tyrosine kinase (PTK) pathway—an important regulator of intracellular signal transduction, representing some of the most frequently occurring mutations found in human malignancies
- The adenomatous polyposis coli (APC) pathway—recognized in oncogenesis pathways
- The glioma-associated oncogene (GLI) pathway—an oncogenesis pathway
- The phosphoinositide 3-kinase (PIK_3) pathway—an oncogenesis pathway
- The SMAD pathway—an oncogenesis pathway
- The hypoxia-inducible transcription factor (HIF)—an oncogenesis pathway
- The retinoblastoma (Rb) pathway—an important cell-cycle regulator
- The P53 pathway—the tumor suppressor protein p53 is inactivated in half of·all human cancers; the p53 pathway interacts with a large number of other signal transduction pathways in a cell; some of these serve as potential therapeutic targets for RNAi intervention
- The apoptosis (APOP) pathway—defects in this pathway are recognized as important to proto-oncogene activation

RNAi has become a powerful laboratory tool to help understand the function of genes and possibly lead to a therapeutic answer for cancer. Favorable results have been found in vitro and in preclinical animal models. Translations to the more complex clinical use are indeed future challenges.

Neurological conditions were once thought to be off-limits to gene therapy approaches because of the blood–brain barrier. However, genetic research activity in this area is progressing. Scientists are investigating the possibility of gene therapy to treat Alzheimer's disease, **epilepsy,** Parkinson's disease, and other neurological diseases.

ALZHEIMER'S DISEASE (AD)

In 1906 Alois Alzheimer, a German physician, peered into the microscope at a slide of brain tissue from of one of his former patients. He had cared for Auguste D. for several years and watched as she progressively lost her mental and physical capabilities. Her behavior went from strange to bizarre; eventually she became completely bedridden and returned to lying in a fetal position. He received permission to do an autopsy and was especially interested in the brain. What he saw shocked him. Her brain was a mass of tangles and deposits he called *plaques.* His question as to the nature of the plaques and tangles, and their relationship to the disease that now bears his name is the subject of the frenzied investigation to halt this disease.

AD is a chronic neurological disorder characterized by the deterioration of the frontal and occipital lobes of the brain. The individual progressively loses memory, language, and the ability to recognize family and friends. Onset is usually between the ages of 40 and 60. According to the Alzheimer's Association, the prevalence rate is about 10.3 percent in persons over 65, and 47.2 percent in those over 85. The time from first symptoms to death may be as long as 20 years.

The hallmarks of the disease are the following:

- Neuroimaging—pictures taken of the brain—reveals that the thinking part of the brain shrinks, ventricles enlarge, and the hippocampus (i.e., the memory chip) loses neurons.
- Microscopic examination reveals deposits outside the neurons of a plaque or deposit of a protein called *B-amyloid,* snipped from a larger protein called *amyloid precursor* (APP). Surrounding the plaques are portions of dying neurons, astrocytes, and microglial cells. Inflammation is also present.
- With the appearance of a collection of tangled threads, neurofibrillary tangles (NFTs) are formed in the nerve cell by the rearranging of microtubules, parts of the cell's internal structure. Normally, the protein called *tau* stabilizes these microtubules, but in AD the microtubules break down and collapse.
- Neurons die, especially in the neocortex.
- Both plaques and NFTs are present in the brains of normal older adults. However, in normal people, the arrangement is not scattered. In persons with AD, the plaque is a compact b-pleated conformation that makes a toxic form.

The Biology of AD

The central problem in AD is recognized as the protein b-amyloid that accumulates and forms plaques in the brain, but how this affects the brain and how it contributes to neurodegeneration are still puzzles. Some researchers have found the specific chemical formula: the 42-amino acid peptide $\alpha\beta$-42. Two accomplices are the enzymes—β-secretase and λ-secretase—that cut out the $\alpha\beta$ from a much larger protein (APP). Genetic studies show that λ-secretase has an active site residing in the protein presenilin-1.

At present, four areas of the genome are known to affect AD:

- Presenilin-1, located on chromosome 14 and suspect for early-onset AD in people at ages 28 to 64
- APP on chromosome 21, for early onset at ages 45 to 64
- Presenilin-2 on chromosome 1, for early onset at age 40 and over
- The gene *APOE* on chromosome 19, identified as a risk factor for AD at ages over 60
- The *PLAU* gene on chromosome 10, which may link plasma A42 to late-onset AD

Other novel suspected regions are on chromosomes 1, 3, 4, 5, 6, 8, 9, 11, 12, 13, 16, 21, and X.

The APOE Gene

The *APOE* gene on chromosome 19 is of special interest. This gene makes a protein called *apolipoprotein E* that combines with fats or lipids in the body and is known as *lipoprotein.* These lipoproteins are responsible for packaging cholesterol and other fats that are carried in the bloodstream and delivered to processing destinations. Three major alleles of the *APOE* gene are the normal form, e3, and two dysfunctional forms, e2 and e4; the most common, e3, is found in at least half of the population. The three isoforms differ only by single-unit amino acids at positions 112 and 158. The gene consists of 50,100,878 to 50,104,489 base pairs and is on the long (q) arm of chromosome 19 at position 13.2 (see Figure 8-1).

The e4 version appears to increase an individual's risk for developing late-onset AD. People who have one copy of the gene have an increased chance of developing AD; those with two copies are at an even greater risk. The *APOE* e4 is associated with an increased number of clumps—the plaques that Dr. Alzheimer saw in Auguste D. However, not all people with AD have the e4 alleles and not all people with e4 develop AD.

Gene Therapy and AD

In 2006 researchers at the Salk Institute and the University of California, San Diego, have used gene therapy to reduce memory loss in mouse models of AD by reducing the amount of an important enzyme β-secretase, or BACE1. According to Oded Singer, one of the authors of the study, mice with AD overcame deficits after progressing to a severe level of the disease. This finding is important because humans are usually not diagnosed until the disease has progressed into recognizable stages. However, amyloid plaques can precede the onset of dementia by many years. Enzymes cut the APP and release toxic fragments that stick together to form clumps. One of the enzymes that damage APP is β-secretase or BACE1.

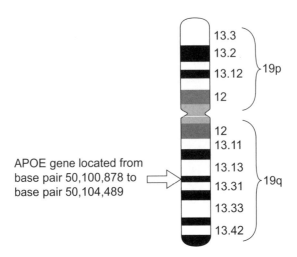

APOE gene located from
base pair 50,100,878 to
base pair 50,104,489

Figure 8-1
The *APOE* gene on chromosome 19.

Traditional gene therapy protocols have sought to introduce normal genes into cells to counteract defective genes. Using RNAi, investigators were able to silence the gene that produces the amyloid plaques. Within a month the mice were able to learn and then to remember their way through a water maze.

Scientists led by Mark Tuszynski at the University of California, San Diego, released a study of the first gene therapy treatment for a patient with AD in 2005 in the journal *Nature Medicine*. First the researchers harvested skin cells from eight patients and inserted the gene that directs the production of a protein called *nerve growth factor* (NGF). NGF is a naturally occurring protein that keeps cells alive and growing in normal brains. Acetylcholine is a neurotransmitter in the brain that assists memory, emotions, and language. Neurosurgeons injected 2.5 million genetically modified cells into the nucleus basalis, a group of cells about the size of the thumbnail at the base of the frontal lobe. After 2 years, positive-emission tomography (PET) scans of patients revealed increased metabolic activity in the brain, a sign of neuron activity. The patients continued to suffer cognitive loss, but at a much slower rate than before gene therapy. This was a phase I safety study.

In 2005 at Rush University Medical Center in Chicago, neurosurgeon Dr. Roy Bakay injected 40 billion viruses into two holes drilled in the head of six patients with mild to moderate AD (see Figure 8-2).

The researchers at Rush used the following procedure:

- They stripped genetic material from the viruses and replaced it with an NGF to keep memory cells alive.
- A computed axial tomography (CAT; now CT) scan located the place where the cells would be injected.

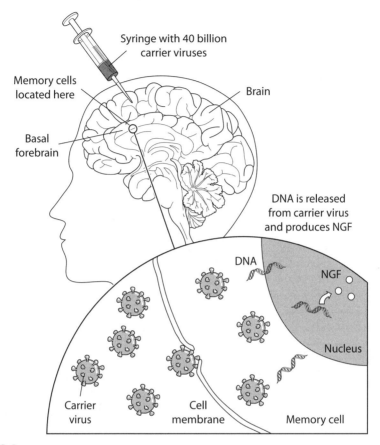

Figure 8-2
Gene therapy for Alzheimer's Disease.

- They located the forebrain, where memory cells are held, and injected it with 40 billion viruses through holes drilled on either side of the upper skull.
- The vector viruses went into the memory cells and released DNA into the nucleus.
- The DNA produced NGF.
- NGF was then released to the rest of the brain to maintain cells important to memory.

EPILEPSY

On 8 November 2006, researchers at the Children's Hospital of Philadelphia announced that they had inhibited the onset of epilepsy after a brain insult in animals. A brain insult is an initial episode of epilepsy or an injury such as a severe head trauma; the patient often develops epilepsy after such insults.

Using gene therapy to modify signaling pathways in the brain, neurology researchers, Amy R. Brooks-Kayal and her colleagues significantly reduced the development of seizures in rats. Seizures are caused by the rapid firing of brain cells and are thought to be caused by an imbalance between the neurotransmitters and the glutamate system, which stimulates neurons to fire, and the neurotransmitter gamma-aminobutyric acid (GABA), which inhibits that brain activity.

Working in a portion of the brain called the *dentate gyrus,* the scientists focused on type A receptors for GABA. GABA(A) receptors are made up of five subunits of proteins that play an important part in brain development and controlling brain activity. Rats with epilepsy had lower levels of the alpha1 subunits of these receptors and higher levels of alpha4 subunits. The researchers used gene therapy to alter the expression of alpha1 subunits and then injected an AD virus carrying the gene that alters the expression of the protein in the brain. Later they injected pilocarpine, a drug that causes status epilepticus (SE), a convulsive seizure. They found that rats that received gene therapy had elevated levels of A1 proteins and either failed to develop seizures or took three times as long to express spontaneous seizure compared to rats that did not receive the gene. According to Brooks-Kayal, this trial shows that there is a window for intervening after a brain insult; it provides proof of the concept that altering signaling pathways in nerve cells after such an insult could provide a scientific basis for prevention of epilepsy.

PARKINSON'S DISEASE (PD)

In 1817 James Parkinson first described a neurological disorder in which patients have shaking tremors in the hands, muscular stiffness, difficulty in balancing and walking, and progressive physical and mental deterioration. The face takes on a frozen, mask-like expression that may become fixed. PD is caused by the death of brain cells that produce a vital chemical known as *dopamine.* A specific area of the midbrain, called the *substantia nigra,* that controls motor coordination is affected. Treatment at present consists of giving a precursor of dopamine, L-Dopa, which can diffuse into the brain. However, over a span of years the medicine becomes less effective.

PD may be a good target for gene therapy for the following reasons:

- Neurological damage is restricted to one area of the brain; this contrasts with AD, in which the entire thinking part of the brain is affected and then the damage spreads to other areas.
- A specific type of cell, the dopamine-producing neuron, is needed to relieve the symptoms of PD.

Researchers experimenting with gene therapy in one PD treatment found long-lasting production of L-Dopa. Using adeno-associated viruses (AAV), researchers delivered two human genes to the specific area of the brain: production was stable for 1 year and there were no observable toxic effects after the treatment.

Genetic research on PD is difficult and inconclusive. Tracing of families with incidents of PD has to concentrate on geographical regions where a condition might have appeared spontaneously in a single individual. The difficulty in this work is that familial cases do not differ from sporadic cases.

Presenting at the Fourteenth Annual Congress of the European Society of Gene Therapy in Athens, Greece, November, 2006, the UK firm Oxford BioMedica released preclinical efficacy data on a gene-based product showing that ProSavin outperformed the standard L-Dopa treatment for PD. Long-term therapeutic benefits showed benefits for at least 15 months without loss of effects. Also, ProSavin does not induce the disabling dyskinesias, or movement disorders, associated with L-Dopa. ProSavin is administered locally to the striatum area of the brain and delivers genes for three enzymes that are required for the synthesis of dopamine. Oxford BioMedica plans to start European phase I and phase II trials in 2007 in patients with late-stage PD, and proposes a clinical plan to follow in a phase III trial, which could begin in 2009.

A different perspective on PD was published in the November 2006 issue of the British journal *Lancet Neurology*. H. C. Fung and colleagues announced that there does not appear to be a gene that strongly influences the risk of PD in most patients, although genes of small influence may still be discovered.

GENETIC DISEASE AND ENVIRONMENTAL FACTORS

Environmental factors, along with genetic propensity for a condition, are important in the development of certain diseases. Lifestyle habits—improper diet, cigarette smoking, and abuse of alcohol and drugs—can activate certain genes.

COLON CANCER

Of the disorders that result from poor diet and habits such as smoking, one of the most obvious is colon cancer. Striking more than 100,000 people each year in North America, this type of cancer results in more than 50,000 deaths annually. Two genes have been identified that make the individual susceptible: the *MSH2* gene located on chromosome 2 and the *MLH1* gene on chromosome 3. If certain environmental conditions are present and the individuals are not living a healthy lifestyle, those carrying mutations of either of these genes may develop colon cancer before the age of 50. Both *MLH1* and *MSH2* code for proteins involved in the repair of DNA. If these repair enzymes are lost or nonfunctioning, multiple mutations may build up, triggering cancer development. Several gene therapy trials are underway.

CARDIOVASCULAR DISEASE

Many types of diseases and disorders can affect the heart and the blood vessels that are part of the cardiovascular system. Scientists are conducting several major gene therapy studies for **atherosclerosis,** a cardiovascular disease affecting the coronary arteries, and for arrhythmias, in which the heart's electrical beating mechanism is abnormal.

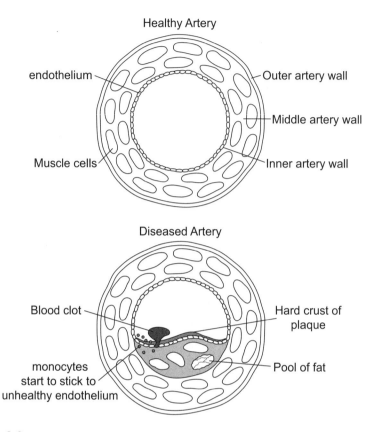

Figure 8-3

Healthy and diseased arteries.

Atherosclerosis, a disease of the arteries, is characterized by a narrowing of the arteries caused by the formation of plaques containing cells and cholesterol. Factors that influence plaque buildup include high levels of cholesterol and triglycerides, high blood pressure, and cigarette smoking. *APOE,* the same gene indicated in Alzheimer's disease, appears to be associated with type III hyperlipoproteinemia, a genetic condition in which lipoproteins—cholesterol, phospholipids, and triglycerides—are increased.

The *APOE* gene sits on the surface of fat particles, including cholesterol and triglycerides, that circulate in the blood. It binds to cells in the liver to rid the body of these fats. The normal version of *APOE,* e3, encoded by a gene on chromosome 19, removes excess cholesterol from the blood by delivering it properly to the liver cells, which store it for later use. The mutant forms of *APOE,* 2 and 4, make proteins that lose the ability to bind to the liver receptors, resulting in buildup of cholesterol in the blood. High blood cholesterol is a major risk factor for coronary heart disease.

A second form of cardiovascular disease affects the arteries of the heart. Coronary arteries carry blood to the cells of the heart muscle, which may die if they become blocked or damaged from the lack of oxygen. The blockage can result in a massive heart attack and death of the patient.

GENE THERAPY FOR HEART DISEASE

Gene therapists are attempting to introduce into the heart a gene that codes for a blood vessel growth factor, to stimulate and repair adequate blood growth. In general, nonviral vectors are not very efficient at delivering genes to cardiovascular cells. Although viruses are more efficient, they have a higher safety risk. Studies in mouse models have revealed that some proteins in the body can help trigger new blood vessel growth and increase the oxygen supply to tissue affected by ischemia, the condition in which blood flow is restricted to an area of the body such as the heart. The blockage is known as *angiogenesis.* These proteins include vascular endothelial growth factor (VEGF) and fibroblast growth factor (FGF).

In February 2000, French scientists transplanted a gene for the human version of *APOE* into mice. The animals had significant reductions in total cholesterol and complete regression from fatty blockages. The most stunning result was found 200 days afterward when plaques in the mice had completely disappeared.

The American Heart Association reported that scientists have used a variety of ways to deliver the genes for VEGF-1 and FGF into humans who suffer advanced myocardial ischemia. After treatment, patients have less severe angina and their hearts function more efficiently. Also, given to patients with limb ischemia, VEGF improved blood supply to the legs and reduced leg sores. Gene therapy with VEGF has improved knee function in some patients for whom amputation appeared to be the only recourse. Gene therapy has been successful in preventing re-occlusion (i.e., re-blockage) of coronary artery bypass grafts, and in keeping arteries open after angioplasty surgery.

Scientists at Rush University Medical Center, Chicago, are studying the use of gene therapy to treat individuals with moderate to severe angina (i.e., chest pain) who have found little relief from traditional medications. This approach grows new blood vessels in the heart. In a phase II trial, VEGF-2 is given in the form of a solution containing DNA plasmids, which is then delivered to the damaged heart tissue via a catheter. The VEGF-2 then stimulates the growth of new blood vessels by promoting growth of endothelial, or lining, cells. The process of growing the new cells, or angiogenesis, occurs within 4 to 8 weeks.

A 2004 study of gene therapy as a substitute for calcium channel blockers, the medication that combats arrhythmias and other forms of heart disease, found a possible alternative to the medication and its side effects. Using guinea pigs, a team from Johns Hopkins University, Baltimore, increased a key protein involved in heart conductivity—G-protein, or Gem—by inserting a virus carrying the gene that codes for the protein into the animal's heart muscles. The effect was similar to that of drugs acting as calcium channel blockers: increased levels of Gem decreased the calcium content density by 30 to 90 percent. When the heart muscle was electrically stimulated to reproduce an irregular heart beat, a Gem infusion steadied the heartbeat, returning it to normal in the same fashion as calcium channel blockers, but without the side effects.

In July 2006 University of Florida researchers released a study discussing a new way of delivering genes with a single injection into a vein. Direct injection into the heart is very inefficient. Barry Byrne and his team found that, by injecting the vector AAV-9 directly into a vein, they could reverse symptoms in mice with a genetic form of Pompe disease, a form of muscular dystrophy that damages the heart. They also tested the virus-based vein delivery method in monkeys and found that heart muscle cells readily absorbed the genes, with the effect lasting for months.

Diabetes Mellitus

Diabetes mellitus is a disease of glucose or sugar metabolism that is defined by high glucose levels in the blood. Three types of diabetes exist:

- Type 1—Insulin-dependent diabetes (IDDM), in which the pancreas does not make enough insulin, the hormone that signals the cells to take up glucose. Studies in twins have shown that the inheritance factor in this type of diabetes is minor. Researchers think that environmental factors and viral antigens are responsible. At one time, this type was called *juvenile diabetes.*
- Type 2—Non-insulin-dependent diabetes (NIDDM). In this type of diabetes, receptors for insulin on the outer surface of target cells do not respond to the presence of glucose. Type 2 is associated with aging and obesity; studies of twins and populations with high incidence of diabetes show a strong genetic component for this type. The gene has been traced to the distal part of the long arm of chromosome 2.
- Gestational diabetes—Only occurs in women during pregnancy.

Several studies are investigating the use of gene therapy as a treatment for diabetes. In 2000 scientists engineered mice to make human insulin in the intestinal cells when they were fed. Normally, only the cells of the pancreas create insulin. The team, based at the University of Alberta, Canada, delivered insulin-making genes into intestinal K cells, which are responsive to blood sugar glucose. They found that the animals were able to make insulin in the intestine and were protected from developing diabetes. When perfected, this procedure could possibly free patients from repeated injections and the complications of diabetes.

One of the problems of delivering genes to treat diabetes is the difficulty of the pancreas as a target. The pancreas is beside the stomach, and the pancreatic structures that produce insulin lie within a remote area, which poses problems in terms of the delivery of gene therapy particles to reach there from the blood. Without a sophisticated way to get the genes to the target, the genes may locate in other body cells and begin to produce insulin, thus causing major problems.

Paul Grayburn and his colleagues at the Baylor University Medical Center in Texas have explored the use of microscopic bubbles that burst with a targeted pulse to deliver insulin genes specifically to the pancreas. They injected the bubbles, which had a shell of water-insoluble molecules, into rats. The bubbles contained a plasmid (i.e., a circular piece) of DNA that coded for a florescent protein marker. When the marker indicated that the plasmid had reached its target in the pancreas, an ultrasonic pulse burst the tiny bubbles, releasing the genetic contents. During dissection, they found high levels of the marker in the pancreatic tissue. A second part of the experiment used bubbles containing plasmids with human genes for insulin.

CARTILAGE REGENERATION

In the April 2006 issue of the *Journal of Bone and Joint Surgery,* Dr. Michael Maloney of the University of Rochester Medical Center, New York, found that light-activated gene therapy treated superficial articular effects and tears in the meniscus. The new procedure is designed to stimulate cartilage regeneration. The research group is hoping to mimic the process in lower vertebrates that regenerates amputated skeletal elements, especially articular cartilage. The controlling set of genes is used only during embryonic development. They found recombinant AAV to be highly efficient at initiating gene therapy in articular chondrocytes. Retreatment with 6000 J/M2, a standard dose of UV light, led to a tenfold increase in the effect of gene therapy in target cells after 1 week. The authors hope this approach might one day be used to treat musculoskeletal disorders, but realize that a number of potential problems with efficacy still exist.

HIV

Gene therapy has also been tested on patients with AIDS. HIV causes AIDS, producing a condition that weakens the immune system so that the person cannot fight off diseases such as certain pneumonias and cancers. Scientists have developed a technique to alter specific HIV proteins to stimulate immune system functioning without causing the negative effects on the system of the complete molecule. Another strategy is to use white blood cells to insert genetically engineered genes, in order to produce a receptor to bind to HIV and reduce its chances of replicating.

In the 1990s scientists found that a number of HIV-positive drug users, who were routinely exposed to HIV, had cellular CCR5 receptors containing genetic mutations that prevent the virus from entering the cell. Researchers from Sangano Biosciences have created genetically modified immune cells that replicate these genetic mutations. Scientists from the company think that this process could potentially provide HIV-positive people with a reservoir of healthy T cells to fight off HIV and opportunistic infections.

In 2006 the private biotechnology corporation VIRxSYS announced the completion of its phase I study of gene therapy. The company's scientists modified the patient's own CD4 T cells—with a virus vector carrying the antisense VRX496—to provide the patient with a number of immune cells capable of resisting HIV infection. The genetically engineered cells repopulated the individual's damaged immune system. Five patients were in the phase I study for 6 months, using the lentiviral HIV, equipped with a genetic medicine containing a long antisense molecule targeted against the HIV envelope gene. The next step is to recruit patients for phase II trials.

PROBLEMS OF SURGERY

Gene therapy may even be used to solve problems associated with surgery. One surgery-related problem occurs in the procedure known as *balloon angio-plasty,* in which a type of scaffold is inserted to open a clogged artery. In response to the foreign object (the scaffold), the body sometimes produces too many cells and causes the artery to reclose, which is called *restenosis.* Gene therapy may prevent this unwanted side effect by covering the outside of the stents used in angioplasty with a soluble gel containing vectors for a gene that reduces the overhealing process.

AGE-RELATED MACULAR DEGENERATION

Oxford BioMedica has developed several lentivirus-based therapeutics for macular degeneration in preclinical and phase I trials.

Although conditions of polygenetic origin are very complicated, many researchers are involved in gene therapy research on a variety of diseases. Some studies are seeking a proof of principle that can be applied to conditions with similar genetic pathways. Gene therapy clinical trials are being conducted around the world to address a variety of diseases. Table 8-2 shows the number of gene therapy trials for specific diseases and conditions.

SECTION TWO

Ethics and Regulations

The year 2001 began the first decade of the new millennium with a cascade of weighty biomedical issues confronting the citizens and government of the modern United States. Other countries also struggled with ethical and regulatory issues. Section Two, consisting of Chapters 9 through 13, considers issues related to the ethics and regulation of gene therapy research. Both sides are presented. Some issues appear in the news media; others are debated only in medical circles. It is not the intent of this book to take a position one way or another but to present perspectives in an unbiased manner.

Issues relating to medical ethics, religion, and regulation are presented. Compelling questions posed in this section include the following:

- What is the meaning of bioethics as it relates to gene therapy?
- What is the likely impact of gene therapy on people's regard for the sanctity of human life?
- What are the risks of inadvertently treating the germ lines?
- How safe must an experiment be before it is ethical to try on humans?
- What alternative methods of treatment are available?
- Is gene therapy likely to be more effective, less costly, or otherwise more acceptable than other available treatments?
- How adequate is the review process that governs gene therapy trials?
- What does informed consent mean for gene therapy trials?
- Do the types of people who volunteer types for gene therapy need addressing?
- Could there be a deliberate misapplication of procedure?

- Are side effects of the treatment reversible or treatable in the patient and in the population?
- Do doctors and scientists have conflicts of interest?

Chapter 9 discusses ethical precepts that must be considered in gene therapy experiments. Chapter 10 presents regulation efforts in the United States, Chapter 11 discusses gene therapy activities in other countries. and Chapter 12 looks at social and religious considerations. Last, Chapter 13 considers future developments and the outlook for gene therapy.

CHAPTER 9

Ethics Issues and Gene Therapy

In *The Boys from Brazil,* a science fiction thriller, Nazi doctors found a way to create 94 clones of Adolf Hitler and sought to have the children raised by parents whose background and occupation would be similar to Hitler's, in hopes of creating another German Führer to revive the Third Reich. In this same spirit, if one were called upon today to write the great science fiction novel devoted to gene therapy, the plot might involve the creation of "designer babies" with certain desirable genes of physical appearance and behavior.

Questions about how gene therapy affects the human race fall under the discipline of ethics, an area of philosophy concerned with what is good and bad and with moral duty and obligation. The word *ethics* comes from the Greek *ethos,* meaning "character." Sometimes the words *ethics* and *morality* are used interchangeably. However, the word *morality* comes from the Latin *moralis,* meaning "customs or manners." Ethics appears to refer to an individual's character, whereas morality is the relationship between human beings.

Ethics also involves the relation of the means to the ends, and in medical research and practice many such dilemmas arise that must be resolved. Medical ethics involves a pattern of values accepted as valid in a particular professional or institutional setting. The ethics are binding on those who belong to a particular group, such as members of the American Medical Association (AMA); sanctions might include loss of the medical license of those who violate the code.

Civil law is related to politics, and differs dramatically from ethical precepts in both scope and sanction. Civil law is binding on all individuals; ethical codes, such as the Hippocratic Oath, apply only to a specific group of people. Individuals who violate civil law face penalties that could include a term of imprisonment, fines, or even capital punishment. Thus, a researcher who violates civil law faces the same courts and penalties as any person who violates the law. For example, the parents of Jessie Gelsinger, the boy who died in a gene therapy experiment, sued in civil court the researchers who conducted the experiment and the university where it was performed.

Medical researchers and professionals are constantly making ethical decisions with major legal implications. Researchers, lawyers, politicians, physicians, theologians, and ethicists must understand key concepts and definitions. In *Issues in American Political Life* (2006), Robert Thobaben et al. list five crucial terms:

1. *Human beings.* Parties involved must agree on what is the essence of life. The idea of consciousness is helpful here. Animals possess consciousness; they react and feel pain. Human beings have self-consciousness. Not only are they aware of circumstances; they are aware that they are aware. This ability to reflect and be aware distinguishes humans from animals and constitutes dignity.
2. *Autonomy.* A human being has the ability to direct one's self, to control one's destiny, and to be responsible for making decisions. In biomedicine, this concept relates to self-direction and personal responsibility.
3. *Informed consent.* The person must be aware of what a procedure will be and must agree to the treatment. The person must be mentally able to make the decision.
4. *Rights.* Two concepts are involved here: moral rights and civil rights. Moral rights are based on one's values and beliefs and are privately revealed to certain individuals, such as family, friends, or trusted physicians. Civil rights are those that are written in legislation or are adjudicated in court decisions.
5. *Malfeasance.* In biomedical issues, a researcher or practitioner may be accused of wrongdoing or misconduct. Medical professionals are morally bound to help others and to do no harm.

ETHICAL ISSUE: FIRST DO NO HARM

When the children who were being treated for ADA developed leukemia, several governments stopped their treatments. However, Great Britain continued the trials, having determined that the risk of the treatment balanced the risk of the children dying from ADA. Such ethical dilemmas face researchers who are considering gene therapy treatments. They must ask the question, will the treatment do harm to a recipient who will die without the treatment?

Where did the idea of "do no harm" originate? It has a long and interesting history. More than 2,000 years ago in Cos, a hilly island off the coast of Greece, Following the Trojan War, Asclepius, the god of medicine, is said to have brought his mortal son Podaios to the island, where all male sons were physicians, known as Asclepiads. Religion and superstition were part of the healing tradition. People came to the holy sites and spent the night in a temple, where the nature of their disease would be revealed to them. The physician-priests then treated the condition, sometimes with extremely harsh treatment. One group of Asclepiads departed from the religious traditions and started a tradition of secular medicine based on observation.

One esteemed practitioner, born about 460 BC, was Hippocrates. He practiced a medicine that was gentle, simple, and often effective. His concern for his patients was paramount, and he wrote in his papers that he would give no deadly medicine to anyone and never injure anyone to benefit another. About 100 AD another Greek physician, Scribonius Largus, refined the writings of Hippocrates into an oath, called the *Hippocratic Oath.* The idea of the oath developed as binding to members of certain professions. For example, physicians take this oath to promise that they will keep a special obligation to patients in their care.

When Europe was plunged into the Dark Ages, physicians were ignorant and untrained, and medical practice involved superstitious nostrums, incantations, and harsh treatment. When the Hippocratic works were found and published during the Renaissance in 1525, institutions began to teach the Hippocratic ideals and required medical practitioners to swear to uphold the oath.

However, for most of history, medical ethics consisted of the individual physician's definition of what was proper conduct. Much has had to do with the inner values of the doctor. A true professional did not feel the need for a formal code, but obviously this approach was subject to a lot of abuse. In 1794 Thomas Percival (1740–1804) of Manchester, England, proposed a code of professional and medical ethics for physicians, for those who worked in hospitals and for the distributors of drugs. When the AMA was founded in 1847, the leaders developed a code similar to Percival's code of ethics. Today, graduates of medical schools take the Hippocratic Oath, in which they pledge not to give a deadly medicine to anyone, even if asked, nor to suggest such council. (See the oath written by Hippocrates in Appendix A.) In addition, the code demands that physicians expose colleagues who are incompetent and who engage in fraud or deception.

KANT'S PRACTICAL IMPERATIVE

During the nineteenth and twentieth centuries, knowledge about medicine was advancing. Many experiments were done on animals, but physicians began to realize that in order to determine whether a treatment would really work, it would have to be tried on humans. Some experiments were done without the consent of the people involved, and some died or were harmed in the trials. For example, during the American Revolutionary War, Hessian prisoners of war were used to test how smallpox was spread. Walter Reed conducted a famous experiment with yellow fever and mosquitoes by assigning half of a group of soldiers to live in barracks without screens while the other half lived in barracks with screens. At the beginning of the twentieth century, some people began to question the ethics of these trials, using the works of German philosopher Immanuel Kant (1724–1804). Kant's ethical principles state that each human being must be considered as a unique end and should never be used as a means to someone else's end. No human being should be used in a trial unless the experiment would be therapeutic for the person involved and would be no more harmful than treatments normally used for such patients. According to Kant's principles, no experimentation for the good of general humanity is acceptable; the individual patient must be the primary beneficiary.

Some ethicists argue that, although this guideline is important, in the instance of patients who realize that they may not benefit personally but that the experiment may advance science and help others, then the treatment is permissible. In this case, the person is fully informed and gives consent for the greater good. These arguments are utilitarian.

ETHICAL ISSUES: HUMAN EXPERIMENTATION AND INFORMED CONSENT

Probably the most pressing ethical issue facing gene therapists is the idea of informed consent. Informed consent is a consequence of the ethical principle of respect for persons. The patient is told about all the possible risks and benefits of a procedure and then weighs the intent, action, and consequences of the decision. Knowing all of the risks and explaining them to patients is a challenge to researchers. Some of the technology is very advanced and complicated. Many genetic procedures are related to children, and a child receiving experimental treatment may not be able to make the decision for him- or herself.

Medical researchers have not always participated in informed consent. The history of medicine reveals some great successes and some horrible abuses. Smallpox, a horrible plague, wiped out entire cities and people were desperate to try anything including experimentation. In 1716 an English aristocrat, Lady Mary Wortley Montagu, heard that ooze from the sores of smallpox victims when scratched into the skin—a process called variolation—gave immunity for some people, and she introduced this practice in England. General George Washington—considering smallpox a more formidable foe than the British—ordered his men to subject to variolation. Some became very ill, some died, but some did not get the disease. It is reputed that Washington forced captured Hessian soldiers to have the test before he would subject his army to it. There was no informed consent here. Washington was severely criticized in Europe for such experiments. When Edward Jenner introduced the idea of using cowpox sores as a vaccine in 1796, he was also vilified.

The Berlin Code was enacted in 1900 when the microbiologist Rudolf Virchow developed a code for experimentation. He realized that only so much could be done with animals and that eventually humans would have to be used to prove whether procedures worked. The Berlin Code was one of the first and strongest of codes governing ethical conditions for use of humans in research. (See the text of the Berlin Code of 1900 in Appendix A.) Unfortunately, Hitler signed a decree in 1931 making the code applicable to Jews, gypsies, persons with mental disabilities, and others. The revelation of Nazi doctors' experiments during World War II drove home the idea of how inhumane and horrible it is to experiment on people without their consent. These revelations led to the Nuremberg Code of 1946.

ETHICAL ISSUE: MALPRACTICE AND MISUSE

The idea of malpractice has already raised its head in genetic treatment. Several lawsuits have been won in cases when doctors failed to fully explain the consequences of giving birth to a child with a genetic disease. When Jesse Gelsinger died, the family sued the University of Pennsylvania on several counts of malpractice. (The complete case *Gelsinger v. University of Pennsylvania* is in Appendix A.) The case was settled out of court for an undisclosed amount.

On the other hand, if the technology of gene therapy ever becomes routine, physicians may one day be sued for failing to treat a genetic disorder. Several questions arise. What should be the standard of care for this technique? Who is responsible? Should only physicians perform gene therapy? Where should it be done? Should all hospitals or only certain ones be designated? Who will make the decisions about those qualified to perform gene therapy?

ETHICAL ISSUE: PATENTS AND TRADE SECRETS

The U.S. Patent Office has determined that genes can be patented; the owner may therefore charge other researchers large sums to use and do experiments on the gene. Is it ethical for this practice of patenting genes to continue? Michael Crichton, physician and author of the best seller *Jurassic Park,* believes this practice is abominable and that procedures or machines should be patented, but not genes. This is tantamount to owning a disease. Crichton believes that such ownerships stymie research and advancement.

ETHICAL ISSUE: INSURANCE

Gene therapy may eventually be covered by standard insurance or it may require special provisions. Cost will certainly enter in. Currently, gene therapy is very expensive; in all likelihood insurance companies will not rush to cover such procedures for their customers.

ARGUMENTS FOR GENE THERAPY

Arguments for and against gene therapy fall into four categories of presentation: teleological, consequential, and utilitarian arguments; deontological or duty-based arguments; arguments from historical precedence; and political arguments.

Teleological, Consequential, and Utilitarian Arguments

The word *teleological* comes from the Greek word *telos,* meaning "end." Consequential and teleological mean the same thing. Utilitarianism is an ethical precept that says that an act is right if it is useful in bringing about a good or desirable end for the greatest number of people. These views are optimistic about gene therapy and support the idea that the end justifies the means of taking risks for the greatest good.

An example of the utilitarian ethical approach came from a 2005 ruling of five Law Lords in the United Kingdom, who determined that families can legally create babies to help sick siblings. The Hasmi family, whose son was born with thalassemia major, claimed that the only hope for their 6-year-old son Zain would be the birth of another child with the same tissue type. The Hasmis had another baby. Doctors took stem cells from the newborn's umbilical cord and transplanted them into Zain. However, other ethicists saw this utilitarian ruling—permitting the creation of "designer babies" for the purpose of therapy—as the beginning of more ominous future actions.

Deontological or Duty-Based Arguments

These arguments propose that gene therapy must be advanced because it is the right thing to do to alleviate human suffering. Some of the genetic diseases are so horrible that humans have a duty to find ways to possibly treat them.

Arguments from Legal and Historical Perspectives

Taking its cue from democracy and majority rule, this argument asserts that, if most of the people approve of a given gene therapy procedure, then the therapy must go forward. It is necessary to move ahead for what is right even though a vocal minority may object.

Political Arguments

The government—with rigid regulators—must support genetic research. If it does not, private rogue activity may take place.

ARGUMENTS AGAINST GENE THERAPY

Teleological objections have been used as arguments against gene therapy. Such objectors, who believe that the end justifies the means and that that end will be good for everyone, do not know what the end will be. They are only guessing. The end may be a brave new world of social engineering, so-called designer babies, or "perfect" people.

Deontological objections have also been used, asserting that the use of some people for the good of other people is morally reprehensible, and that it is the duty of humans to respect all humans for their own unique value.

Slippery-slope arguments argue against gene therapy as well. Once gene therapy comes into accepted use, no one knows where it will end. Treating diseases may lead to changing the genome and to the slippery slope of getting more than what was anticipated.

Others who argument against gene therapy are concerned with the scientists. Are scientists to be trusted? Are they developing data and keeping them secret to build their egos? In the Gelsinger case, the researchers who were involved were charged with having monetary interest in the success of the experiments. A University of Michigan researcher published a study in 2006 that echoed this sentiment. He cites a dozen incidents each year of serious misconduct that question the integrity of science.

Human gene therapy experimentation raises many issues. Although the promise of the technology is very great, in reality it is also very dangerous. These ethical questions are only the beginning as gene therapy continues to develop over the years. The arguments are similar to those advanced for and against any cutting edge technology, such as stem cell research and nanotechnology. However, ethical questions lead to the obvious conclusion: there must be regulations. Chapter 10 addresses the development of these regulations.

CHAPTER 10

Regulatory Actions in the United States

Will natural blondes go extinct in 200 years? Were Neanderthals smarter than we are? Are modern Americans, infantilized by higher education, incapable of growing up? Michael Crichton, author of *The Andromeda Strain* and *Jurassic Park*, has penned a new novel called *Next*, based on genetic manipulation. In the novel, cancer survivor Frank Burnet discovers that the cells he allowed a doctor to harvest from his body were sold for research to a private firm named Biogen. When the expensive cells become contaminated, the company claims to have rights to take the cells by force from Burnet. Burnet hides, and a bounty hunter kidnaps his daughter and granddaughter, who also have the valuable genes. In the meantime in other parts of the world, an orangutan with human genes curses tourists in Sumatra, and a parrot named Gerard embarrasses people by making illicit sounds. A donor to a sperm bank finds out that his sperm was used to create a transgenic chimpanzee, whom he eventually adopts and to whom bullies at school give the nickname, "Monkey boy."

Crichton has created a fanciful and intriguing plot where all the elements come together. When he speaks about his work at book signings, he acknowledges that the story is fantasy. However, he foresees that, if genetic manipulation is not controlled in time, possibly the slippery slope will come about as it is portrayed in these scenes. He offers several policy recommendations for the regulation of genetic research, which include banning the patenting of genes, banning certain types of germ-line research, and establishing clear guidelines for the use of human tissues.

Few initiatives in health care have generated more excitement than gene therapy. As discussed in Chapters 5 through 8, gene therapy holds promise for not only treating but also for curing diseases such as cancer, diabetes, and cystic fibrosis. Although the scenarios in *Next* will probably never happen, Chapters 5 through 8 illustrate how much remains unknown about gene therapy. Scientists do not know the short- and long-term risks that are involved. Thus, the

challenge to the gene therapy community is to balance the risks with the therapeutic benefits. Their challenge is like a balance scale. On one side, scientists
must weigh and predict the actual risks based on factors that may be unknown,
and balance these risks with the benefit to patients who have diseases with no
cure. The drawing of the balance in Figure 10-1 is simple, but when all the factors are added on piece by piece, the process becomes tedious and slow.

Numerous agencies of the federal government oversee the development and
application of human gene therapy in the United States: the FDA, the NIH, the
Center for Biologics Evaluation and Research (CBER), the Office of Biotechnology Activities (OBA), the Recombinant DNA Advisory Committee (RAC), and
the Office of Human Subjects Research (OHSR). Involving so many groups,
committees, and agencies, the process of regulating and legislating gene therapy
is very complex. In addition, the courts may be involved in civil or criminal
issues that need to be resolved.

FOOD AND DRUG ADMINISTRATION

Gene therapy involves the treatment of a patient. Because the procedure is
delivered through various vectors, the treatment is considered a drug, and so its
ultimate approval and oversight are the responsibility of the FDA. The FDA, an
agency under the Department of Health and Human Services (HHS), has eight
centers and offices that regulate all aspects of food, drugs, and technology. Its mission is to promote and guard public safety by making sure that approved drugs are
safe and effective.

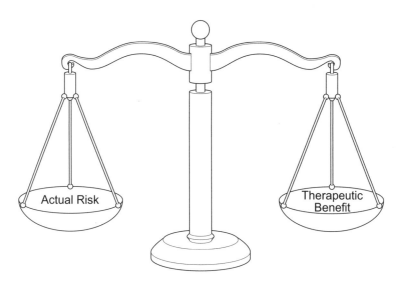

Figure 10-1
The balance of risk versus benefit.

Between 1750 and 2000, health care evolved from the simple use of home remedies and treatment by itinerant doctors to a scientific and technical complex, supervised and highly regulated. In 1862 the FDA had one chemist to analyze and test the safety of food. Responding to the ease with which quacks and charlatans could peddle unsafe and useless potions, Congress passed the Pure Food and Drug Act in 1906. The agency was expanded in 1936 when the Federal Food, Drug, and Cosmetic Act gave power to the courts to prosecute violators. The FDA was positively recognized in the 1950s when a director kept thalidomide from being approved, and saved American children from having to live with the sort of deformities that more than 12,000 babies in Europe were born with. In 1962 the Kefauver Amendments were added to the Food, Drug, and Cosmetic Act to ensure greater drug safety. For the first time, drug manufacturers were required to prove to the FDA that products were safe and effective before marketing them.

In 1984 the FDA created CBER, which regulates gene therapy. In 1991 CBER issued a document that spelled out the precautions required to be taken in manufacturing and testing gene therapy products. Unlike drugs, biologics—treatments derived from humans, animals, or microorganisms—are very complex; many of them are manufactured using biotechnology and genetic engineering. The DNA and viral vectors used in gene therapy are products that the FDA must regulate, licensing the gene therapy trials through CBER.

To begin a review for use of a new therapy, the researchers are required to follow a tedious process. First, the Investigational New Drug (IND) application subjects the study to great scrutiny. An IND review team is assigned, consisting of the following individuals:

- A product reviewer
- A pharmacology and toxicology reviewer
- A clinical reviewer
- A regulatory project manager
- A consulting reviewer (if needed)

The emphasis in the IND review process is on data. Documents must show that the product is safe, that manufacturing and quality control issues are sound, and that the protocol has scientific rationale. The rationale is established during preclinical studies and through product development procedures and sound clinical protocols. In addition to following this procedure, which is required with all drugs, gene therapy involves consideration of three unique issues:

- The potential for rescue of replicating virus
- The potential for permanent alteration to somatic or germ-line DNA, and for long-term toxicity
- Consideration of enhancement (which simply makes something better) versus treatment (which could be therapy, or possibly a cure)

If the license is given, CBER receives regular reports and conducts routine on-site investigations.

In 1993 a serious adverse event (SAE) that was linked to an AD virus vector in a trial prompted the FDA to release a guidance document for the regulation of gene therapy. The document defined gene therapy as a medical procedure based on genetic modification of living cells, and asserted that genetic manipulation is designed to treat disease or injuries in humans.

Following the development of leukemia in X-SCID patients in trials in France, the FDA tightened its demands upon researchers in October, 2002, to include the following requirements:

- Revised informed consent documents
- Plans for monitoring patient samples for vector integration every 6 months for the first 5 years and then annually for the next 10 years
- For certain experiments, a second test within 3 months of the first, with the sequence analyzed and the subject monitored closely for signs of malignancy

NATIONAL INSTITUTES OF HEALTH

The NIH began in one room as a laboratory of hygiene in 1887. Congress allocated $35,000 in 1901 to fund a new agency, the Public Health and Marine Service Hospital. A new building to house it in Washington DC, was completed in 1904. In 1912 another law shortened the agency's name to Public Health Service, and then in 1930 it was renamed the National Institute of Health. When cancer became a problem of interest, the Senate voted to fund the National Cancer Institute (NCI) and built a campus in Bethesda. In 1944 the NCI became part of the NIH and the word "Institute" became plural—the National Institutes of Health—in 1948.

In 1974 the NIH established the Office of Biotechnology Activities (OBA), which then formed the Recombinant DNA Advisory Committee (RAC). The RAC is charged with recommending safe guidelines for research involving rDNA. In 1980 the OBA shifted its focus from rDNA to a newly devised procedure known as gene therapy. The RAC formed the Working Group on Human Gene Therapy, which consisted of scientists, clinicians, lawyers, ethicists, policy experts, and public representatives. The Working Group provided a list of questions that researchers must address in submission to the RAC. All protocols funded by the NIH must be submitted to the RAC for approval; however, a clinical trial cannot proceed until the FDA has approved it. Thus, both organizations have responsibility for monitoring NIH-funded trials. Trials funded only by pharmaceutical or biotechnology companies need only the approval of the FDA. The RAC has made it clear that it will not fund germ-line transfer experiments.

The NIH monitoring effort is the responsibility of the OBA, to which the RAC belongs. If these overseers discover a breach in regulations, law requires them to report it to the FDA, which can then terminate trials and order investigations.

In April 2002 the NIH guidelines were released. (Appendix A includes the text of the *Guidelines for Research Involving Recombinant DNA Molecules*.) The guidelines are written in "legalese" and are difficult to follow, filled with cross-references, exceptions, lists, sections, appendices, and tables. However abstruse, they are binding on researchers.

Each institution has an Institutional Biosafety Committee (IBC) called the Committee on Microbial Safety (COMS). The NIH requires all laboratories working with rDNA to register with their IBC. The NIH's OBA is the administrative arm responsible for carrying out the orders with regard to rDNA, genetic testing, and xenotransplantation. An advisory committee is involved in establishing policies for each of these fields. For rDNA, the committee is the RAC.

All human gene transfer protocols are currently considered experimental. COMS approval must await RAC action. Depending on whether the study is deemed novel, the RAC can schedule a full examination of the protocol at one of its quarterly meetings or recommend sole FDA review. Overcoming the regulatory hurdles in gaining approval for a human gene transfer study is not for the faint of heart. Beyond approval from the FDA comes approval from the Biosafety Committee of the local Institutional Review Board (IRB). Also, the NIH RAC evaluates novel protocols although it does not have approval power. These evaluations often involve the appearance of the principal investigator (PI) for aggressive questioning by members of the RAC. This intimidating procedure is usually addressed by use of a specialized consultant or a commercial sponsor. Once approved, the PI must make regular reports to the NIH. A report is due within 20 working days of the first subject enrollment. At the 1-year anniversary of the FDA's IND approval, a report similar to the FDA annual reports is sent to the NIH. Any SAEs must be reported within 15 days.

To assist in managing gene therapy, the FDA and the NIH launched the Genetic Modification Clinical Research Information System (GeMCRIS) in 2004. This database on gene therapy gives the public information about ongoing clinical trials and encourages the reporting and analysis of SAEs related to these trials.

When Jesse Gelsinger died in 1999 from unexpected complications of his gene therapy, the case received national media attention and spurred efforts for closer collaboration among all involved in the field.

To make sure that all bases are covered, the FDA and NIH have complementary responsibilities relating to gene therapy. Both agencies review proposed gene therapy studies. The process of submitting for trials is very complex and involves a great amount of data from preclinical studies. The FDA's primary role is to ensure that manufacturers produce safe gene therapy products and that the protocols for human subjects are properly followed. The primary job of the NIH is to evaluate the quality of science and to fund studies deemed to advance the technology and tools of clinical studies.

GeMCRIS is an educational effort to enable patients, researchers, scientists, product sponsors, and the public to become better informed about gene therapy research. Information is available about what trials are being conducted, where they are being conducted, and what investigational approach is being used. Monitoring SAEs for trials is extremely important. This collaborative effort involves the two agencies working together.

The FDA has not approved any gene therapy products yet, but numerous clinical studies may meet the standards. The Web site for GeMCRIS is www.gemcris.od.nih.gov.

INSTITUTIONAL REVIEW BOARDS AND INFORMED CONSENT

From 1932 to 1972, the U.S. Public Health Service conducted syphilis research on indigent black men. Researchers withheld treatment from the men in order to study the natural progression of the disease. In July 1974, revelations about these experiments led to adoption of the National Research Act (P.L. 93-348), which added restrictions and oversight procedures for research involving human subjects. The Commission for the Protection of Human Subjects of Biomedical and Behavioral Research issued the Belmont Report (named for the Belmont Conference Center at the Smithsonian Institution, where the commission met). Appendix A includes the text of the Belmont Report.

The Belmont Report includes the following points:

- All human subjects of research should be treated with respect shown to persons as individuals.
- Human research subjects should never be injured for the benefit of others.
- Volunteers must receive some benefit from their participation.
- All persons must consent in writing to the experimental treatment and receive information in a way that they can understand.
- Volunteers must be aware of the risks and benefits.
- Subjects must be selected in a fair manner. High-risk experiments that use prisoners or low-income people as subjects are not acceptable.

The Belmont Report introduced the principle of informed consent; the FDA and NIH are responsible for checking its guidelines. Local groups, or institutional review boards (IRBs), must review the protocols that govern use of human subjects. To win approval to conduct trials, a protocol is required to pass through many reviews.

PRIVATE VOICES

The government is not the only voice concerned about quality in the field of gene therapy. The U.S. Pharmacopeia (USP) is a nongovernmental group that is independent, not-for-profit, and self-supporting. The USP seeks to promote public health by establishing and disseminating officially recognized standards of quality and authoritative information for use by both professionals and consumers. The USP uses volunteer committees of experts from academia, industry, and the government. In the 1995–2000 revision cycle, an advisory panel for biotechnology was formed to review the field of gene and cell therapy. The panel recommended ways and means to provide practitioners with clear information about the emerging field, and in June 2005 began working on developing that document for review.

COURTS

In the United States, two kinds of courts—criminal and civil—make rulings that affect the development of policy and law. A case is tried in criminal court when an individual breaks a law or statute and the state is the plaintiff. (The accuser is the plaintiff and the accused is the defendant.) Those who perceive that another person or organization has wronged them may seek to have the case adjudicated in a civil court. The plaintiff seeks to right the wrong through action, or possibly through the award of monetary damages.

THE JESSE GELSINGER LEGAL TRIAL

Background of the Case

Jesse Gelsinger, an 18-year-old Arizona teenager, had a rare condition—ornithine transcarbamylase (OTC) deficiency—which affected his cells' ability to get rid of ammonia. He was able to control this condition with diet and drugs—32 pills a day. The protocol that he volunteered for had no chance of providing him—or any other volunteer—with any benefit. Before the gene therapy trial, the researchers at Pennsylvania determined the following:

- The protocol was designed only to test the safety of a treatment that would be used for babies with OTC deficiency. The scientists believed that OTC deficiency could be surmounted with gene therapy.
- They hoped to infuse babies with OTC deficiency with a gene that would help them produce the missing enzyme.
- To get these genes into the cells, researchers developed a weakened cold virus, the AD virus, to deliver the corrected OTC gene.
- The procedure would control the high levels of ammonia in babies with OTC deficiency immediately after birth.

Jesse was deemed eligible and was assigned to a group of subjects who received the highest dose of the AD virus. The doctors thought that the worst-case scenario would result in an inflamed liver, which could be treated. They were totally unprepared for Jesse's death on 17 September 1999.

Jesse's family sued the university in civil court. The defendants were the trustees of the University of Pennsylvania; Dr. James Wilson and his company, Genovo, Inc.; and attending physicians Steven Raper and Mark Batshaw. Arthur Caplan, an ethicist at the University of Pennsylvania, was also named in the suit because of advice he had given the other defendants. The details of the counts in the case are given in Appendix A. The suit's basic counts cited

- *Wrongful death.* The defendants were careless and reckless in their conduct and failed to properly assess the suitability of admitting Jesse to the trial.
- *Survival.* In causing the death, the defendants kept Jesse from the earnings he would have made during his lifetime.
- *Product liability.* Researcher Dr. James Wilson was the founder and one of the owners of the biotech company that manufactured the AD virus used in the trial. The product was poorly tested.
- *Lack of informed consent.* The defendants did not warn Jesse of all of the risks.
- *Misleading information.* The defendants did not give correct and complete information to Jesse and therefore caused him to suffer emotional distress.

- *Fraud on the FDA.* The team deliberately made false misrepresentations to the FDA.

The University of Pennsylvania settled out of court for an undisclosed amount.

Jesse's death forced government officials to reappraise the framework and structure of gene therapy research and to reexamine informed consent procedures. They were also forced to take public responsibility for their action.

Although the procedures of regulation outlined in this chapter are complex and confusing, the U.S. government seeks to assure that it approves only ethical and responsible research. Human gene therapy must be seriously and cautiously evaluated. Chapter 11 considers some of the procedures and regulations in place in other countries—which may not be as rigorous.

CHAPTER 11

Gene Therapy in Other Countries

When 62-year-old Hashmukh Patel realized that traditional chemotherapy in the United States was not going to kill the cancerous tumor in his esophagus, he made his way to Beijing, China for an injection of a gene therapy drug called Gendicine. This treatment is not available in the United States, but it is the first commercial gene therapy drug, available only in China, at a cost of $20,000 for a 2-month treatment. Patel is only one of the 70 foreign patients from 22 countries who have sought this treatment.

When the *Gelsinger* case and other failed cases caused major setbacks in the West, Chinese researchers saw the opportunity to take ideas originated in the United States and make them work. For example, SiBono Gene Tech Co. in Shenzhen developed its drug Gendicine, which is similar to a gene therapy treatment created by Introgen Therapeutics in Austin, Texas. Gendicine uses the *p53* gene, which suppresses tumor formation with a modified virus. When the product is injected into a tumor, the virus carries the gene to the cancer cells, which then "commit suicide." China does not have the same regulatory procedures for the development of drugs that other countries do.

On 9 February 2006, China's State Council announced that biotechnology research would be a top priority, and committed to spending 2.5 percent of the gross domestic product to research and development. Many of the researchers were trained in the United States and then returned to China. The father of China's gene therapy is Peng Zhaohui, who worked at the UCLA medical school and at a biotechnology start-up in San Diego in the mid-1990s. Peng believes that China is an ideal place to work because more than 2 million Chinese citizens are diagnosed with cancer every year. The cost of clinical trials is about one-tenth the cost in the United States and the regulatory climate is favorable. The government is more open to innovation than are the FDA and counterparts in the United States. The Chinese acknowledge that there are risks to gene therapy, but also acknowledge the risks to surgery, radiation, and chemotherapy.

In different countries, the development of regulations related to gene therapy differ. In the United States, the guidelines are very complicated and the hoops to jump through are many for scientists who seek approval (see Chapter 10, Regulatory Actions in the United States). Countries in the West, such as the United Kingdom and European Union, have similar codes. However, the developing countries, especially in the Far East, do not impose stringent regulations.

Regulatory procedures first arose abroad, beginning in the United Kingdom. Issues related to in vitro fertilization and cloning were addressed in 1978 with the formation of the Human Fertilization and Embryology Authority. In 1990 the United Kingdom enacted the Human Fertilization and Embryology Act, which governed fertility and stem cell research. In 1993 the Gene Therapy Advisory Committee (GTAC) was formed to review proposals and make recommendations to the Department of Health. One major function of the committee is to see that the protocols of research are carried out according to the Nuremberg and Belmont agreements.

The GTAC is the UK national research ethics committee for gene therapy clinical research, according to the Medicine for Human Use (Clinical Trials) Regulations 2004, article 5. The GTAC must agree to all somatic research before trials can begin. Under Clinical Trials Regulations, the GTAC is required to provide an ethical opinion on applications for use of products within 90 days of receipt of a valid application. The GTAC's definition of gene therapy includes techniques such as the following for delivering synthetics or recombinant nucleic acids into humans:

- Genetically modified biological vectors such as viruses or plasmids
- Genetically modified stem cells
- Oncolytic or cancer-causing viruses
- Nucleic acids associated with delivery vehicles
- Naked nucleic acids
- Antisense techniques, such as gene silencing, gene correction, and gene modification
- Genetic vaccines
- DNA or RNA technologies such as RNAi
- Xenotransplantation of animal cells (but not animal organs)

In 1992 the Clothier Committee on the Ethics of Gene Therapy recommended that gene therapy be conducted on diseases that are life-threatening, but not be used for germ-line research. The GTAC takes into account the scientific merits and potential benefits of gene therapy versus the risks.

In April 2005 the GTAC announced the details of 11 gene therapy trials that have been approved. The majority of the studies focus on cancer, including colorectal cancer, prostate cancer, leukemia, brain cancers, breast cancer, and advanced tumors. Three trials are for coronary heart disease and one represents an approach to combat HIV. The report also included all 96 UK trials carried out to that date. The GTAC states that the United Kingdom leads Europe in gene therapy trials.

EUROPEAN UNION

The European Union includes 14 countries on the continent of Europe plus Ireland. Other countries' requests to join the European Union are pending. The group that supervises gene therapy, the European Agency for the Evaluation of Medicinal Products (EMEA), is the centralized regulatory organ for the evaluation of quality, safety, and efficacy of medicinal products, including gene therapy. The Council Regulation 2309/ED adopted by the European Council of Ministers in July 1993 established the legal basis of operation of the EMEA.

All gene therapy products must be authorized through a centralized procedure, and researchers must submit an application dossier similar to that for all other medicinal products. The EMEA basically agrees with the policies of GTAC.

ASIA

This chapter began with a story about a gene therapy trial in China that could not possibly be done in the United States or in any other Western country. Several Asian countries have developed aggressive attitudes about cutting-edge research in stem cells, cloning, and gene therapy. Much of the original research is done in Western countries, but it cannot be carried into trials because of the rigid procedures. In February 2004 Woo Suk Hwang announced in the journal *Science* that his team had cloned 30 embryos and harvested stem cells from one of them. Biologists throughout the world began to worry that Asia was ahead of the West and was winning the battle for cutting-edge science. Hwang attributed his success to the supportive environment of South Korea's well-funded laboratories and legislation that was supportive of cutting-edge experimentation. However, trouble lurked around the corner. The Seoul-based Munhwa Broadcasting Corporation challenged the credibility of his studies. Later investigations revealed that large amounts of data in the studies were fabricated. Hwang had been considered a national hero in Korea, but he was later charged with fraud, embezzlement, and faked research. The government revoked his license in spring 2006 and barred him from conducting cloning experiments or receiving human eggs for research. Hwang still claims that he created the first cloned human stem cells.

Undaunted by this scandal over research, South Korean scientists are continuing work in the area of genetic research. Lee Byung-chun, who was denied the right to teach students for 5 months because of his contributions to a paper written by Hwang, is continuing his investigative work on dogs. Korean scientists created the successfully cloned dog, Snuppy, an Afghan hound, and they recently cloned three female puppies for reproductive purposes. Their focus is on manipulating dogs' genes so that they will have the same diseases as those affecting humans and will be useful for gene therapy experiments. In December 2006 Chang Kyu-tae announced that the state-funded Korean Research Institute for Bioscience and Biotechnology had given approval for a project to clone a monkey by the end of 2009. The scientists believe that monkeys, who are closer to human biology than other animals, would be more reliable for developing techniques such as gene therapy or for growing new organs using stem cells.

ISRAEL

The Israeli National Knowledge Center for Gene Therapy at the Goldyne Savad Institute of Gene Therapy supports and motivates researchers in Israel with funding from the Israel Ministry of Science. The Center's goal is to provide researchers with tools to help them overcome major obstacles in the process. To assist in dissemination of knowledge to the scientific and medical community and to facilitate the progress of gene therapy projects, Israel has established the following units:

- Viral vector construction unit—This unit helps investigators build viral vectors and gather knowledge about naked DNA delivery methods such as hydrodynamic injection and electroporation. Planned for the future is a laser beam gene transfer system.
- Imaging unit—This unit helps develop the effectiveness of delivery systems. At present, it provides cutting-edge imaging systems, including a system that monitors luciferase expression, a detection camera to monitor green fluorescent protein (GFP) expression, and the Cell Vizio system to detect low-level and single-cell expression of fluorescently expressed proteins in vivo. In addition, the unit assists with fMRI monitoring and ultrasound imaging.
- Pharmacogenomic unit—This unit tailors preferred regulatory elements to each specific expression system to be used in gene therapy. For any given project, the promoters and enhancers are selected using this computerized bioinformatics tool.
- GMP production rooms—Rooms are provided for investigators to produce their delivery systems in an approved environment with investigators who can give technical advice. The unit provides support in drafting their standard operation procedures and in performing their studies.

Globalization is relevant to the area of gene therapy. The first regulated studies were performed in the United States in the mid-1990s. Since then more than 7,000 patients have been treated in more than 1,000 studies spanning 15 countries across several continents (as listed in Table 11-1).

Likewise, various modalities of gene therapy are used to treat a variety of diseases (see Table 11-2).

Table 11-1   Distribution of Gene Therapy by Continent

Continent	Number of Trials	Percentage of Total Trials
North and South America	790	67
Europe, including UK and EU	338	29
Asia	32	2.7
Australia	19	1.6
Africa	1	0.1

Adapted by Evelyn B. Kelly from information in *The Journal of Gene Medicine,* updated July 2006.

Table 11-2 Modalities of Gene Therapy Used in Trials

Gene Type	Number of Trials
Cytokine	312
Antigen	189
Tumor suppressor	139
Suicide	94
Deficiency	72
Drug resistance	56
Replication inhibitor	45
Receptor	44
Antisense	9
Oncogene regulator hormone	8
Marker	6
Hormone	6
Ribozyme	6
Others	168
Unknown	38
Total	1192

Adapted by Evelyn B. Kelly from the *The Journal of Gene Medicine,* updated July 2006.

Table 11-3 Countries Participating in Gene Therapy Clinical Trials

Country	Number of Gene Therapy Clinical Trials
USA	775
UK	136
Germany	73
Switzerland	42
France	19
Belgium	19
Australia	17
Japan	15
Italy	15
Canada	13
Netherlands	12
Israel	6
China	4
Norway	4
South Korea	4
Spain	4
Poland	3
Finland	3
Singapore	2
New Zealand	2
Austria	2

(Continued)

Table 11-3 *(Continued)*

Country	Number of Gene Therapy Clinical Trials
Denmark	2
Sweden	2
Czech Republic	1
Mexico	1
Russia	1
Taiwan	1
Multicountry	12
Total	1192

Adapted by Evelyn B. Kelly from the *The Journal of Gene Medicine,* updated July 2006.

As of July 2006, about 1,192 projects were in progress throughout the world. In the United States, 776 trials were in process or in review by the RAC of the NIH. More than 28 countries are experimenting with gene therapy (listed in Table 11-3).

Two gene therapy agents are available on the market: Fomiversan, an antisense construct for the treatment of cytomegalovirus retinitis in AIDS patients, and the *p53* tumor suppressor gene for treating patients with cancer of the head and neck, for whom therapy is available only in China. A large number of the patients in the first gene therapy trials were administered marker genes, not therapeutic genes. Out of the thousands treated, two deaths have been attributed directly to gene therapy. These mortality rates are low compared to mortality statistics for chemotherapy and transplantation.

CHAPTER 12

Social and Religious Issues

Is designing a baby with a defect unethical? Many of the religious reservations expressed about human gene therapy refer only to alterations that might affect the germ line to produce inherited changes. But what if the parents have some type of defect and want a child with the same defect? According to a 22 December 2006 news story, four clinics in the United States are reported to have provided the costly, complicated procedure to help families create children with a disability. Cara and Gibson Reynolds of Collingswood, New Jersey, are "little people" (i.e., dwarfs), who desire to have a child who is like them. A story in the online magazine *Slate* headlined "Old Fear: Designer Babies. New Fear: Deformer Babies" termed this the "deliberate crippling of children." When the story was published, the Reynoldses were outraged at the opposition to using embryo screening to allow dwarf couples to have dwarf children. Although the *Slate* story related to preimplantation genetic diagnosis (i.e., embryo screening), genetic manipulation could also eventually be involved. The story challenges us to think of making not only children who are perfect, but also children who are chosen to have a disability.

This scenario creates a world of social and religious implications. Will gene therapy lead down the slippery slope of creations that society cannot handle? Currently, most social and religious groups accept gene therapy more than other cutting-edge research, such as stem cell research and nanotechnology. According to a 1984 perspective from the World Council of Churches, gene therapy that is restricted to only somatic cell corrections of single-gene traits is viewed as little different from other medical therapies. In a democratic society of religious freedom, different social groups may react differently. However, gene therapy does not generally excite religious controversy. Because it involves the destruction of embryos for research and arouses the specter of abortion, embryonic stem cell research provokes opposition among some religious groups; but this is not the case with gene therapy.

SOCIAL ISSUES

Applying gene therapy to human suffering is most likely to be regarded by society as a significant step. Most of the differences between gene therapy and other medical procedures are perceptual. The risks are the same as for such other therapies as pharmaceutical intervention, surgery, and radiation. The social aspects of gene therapy fall into three categories:

- What process determines who needs gene therapy and when to begin it?
- How important are evolutionary considerations?
- What will be the impact on social institutions?

What Process Determines Who and When?

One of the arguments raised after the Gelsinger death was that Jesse was not a good candidate and should never have been in the experiment. He was not sick before he died and his condition, OTC deficiency, was being controlled with a low-protein diet and 32 pills a day. He knew when he signed up that he would not benefit and that it was a phase I study to test a treatment for babies with a fatal form of the disease. This is an illustration of an ethical dilemma. Who should get gene therapy and who decides when it should begin? Some judgments are technical, but others involve such decisions as quality of life. Should Jesse have accepted a lifetime regimen of 32 pills a day and a diet so restrictive that eating half a hot dog was considered a treat? Jesse, his parents, and the researchers made the decision. It turned out to be a bad one.

The answer to this question is made in the context of a particular family and particular children. When several children developed leukemia as a result of the SCID-X1 test, gene therapy experiments were halted in several countries. However, experimentation was allowed to continue in the United Kingdom because there had been some UK successes, and some children had died from the natural disease while waiting for the procedure. The reality is that different people react to treatment in different ways. Determining the risks is not an exact science.

In considering who will make the decisions, some urge caution in approaching gene therapy in general. In 1984 Jeremy Rifkin posed the slippery slope argument: once the process of genetic engineering begins, there is no logical place for it to stop. The scenario of the "little people" (dwarfs) who wanted a child who shared their own disability is one example. Although scientists may help us gain health, is it worth trading our humanity for? Ola Huntley (1983) pleaded for support for gene therapy to treat conditions like sickle cell disease. Her three children have this disease, and she described the human agony of their suffering. She asked the question: Who should deny these children and others like them the right to essential genetic treatment for their disease? These two conflicting points of view represent two sides of the social implications of gene therapy.

Social scientists who study public policy have these same ethical questions raised in the context of other medical interventions, such as the administration of antibiotics or the acceptance of surgery. Policy has to be based on such considerations as patient welfare, social impacts, religious precepts, and political realities.

Obviously, government agencies must be involved in decisions about gene therapy because of their involvement in medical research, health care, and issues that attract wide public interest.

How Important Are Evolutionary Considerations?

Discussion of germ-line gene therapy is most relevant to permanently changing the human gene pool because it could lead to inherited changes. At present, speculation about germ-line changes is vague and seems unreal. However, with advances in technology, this aspect may become reality. Scientists can create new arrangements of genes, implant them into a bacterium, and watch the new bug reproduce and divide. A huge problem arises in that changing the genetic code of human beings alters the genetic constitution of people and is thus a momentous step. Who decides to do this? Are scientists obliged to defer to a parent who wants a child with blonde hair, blue eyes, and musical talent? Are they obliged to create for parents with a disability such as dwarfism, a child with the same disability? What traits should be emphasized? How is it possible to know the long-term effects of such manipulations seven generations from now?

Recombinant genetic technologies permit genes from one species to be inserted into another. Human genes are used in animals to test the safety and efficacy of gene therapy. Some people fear that animal genes will be used in humans.

What Will Be the Impact on Social Institutions?

Will the focus of society turn from humanity to mechanistic interpretations? The specific effect of gene therapy in changing perceptions may become related to that in other fields that challenge self-perception, such as neuroscience, computer science, psychology, evolutionary biology, ecology, and other areas of biology and medicine.

Gene therapy may play a larger role in altering parental expectations. More parents may expect "perfect children." As long as gene therapy is confined to diseases that are recognized as burdens, the area is like other medical treatments. However, if attempts are made to affect intelligence or physical traits, this could open a slippery slope. With technology advancing every day, discussion about these issues needs to be encouraged.

RELIGIOUS IMPLICATIONS

Most of the discussion about genetic enhancement is rooted in the Judeo-Christian tradition on the religious side, and in the Hippocratic Oath and other Western philosophical traditions on the secular side.

Christian Traditions

Although great diversity and pluralism exists among both Catholics and Protestants, the churches generally share the common thread of divine revelation in the person of Jesus, the goodness of creation, and the need for compassion and justice. Religious questions about genetic manipulation fall into three categories:

the possibility of humans playing God, the meaning of "being human," and the need to respect human life.

Are Humans Playing God?

The question is often asked whether it is right for human beings to manipulate human genes at all. Are humans, in a sense, playing God by altering fundamental aspects of the makeup of humans, plants, and animals, which is the prerogative of God alone? Is it dangerous to tamper with nature in ways in which humans have neither the right nor the skill? In manipulating human genes, are people playing God?

Donald Bruce of the Church of Scotland responds that most Christian believers have viewed scientific research as a proper response to God's commands to "fill the earth and subdue it" and to "work and take care of" the garden. This refers to the picture of Adam in the Garden of Eden as he was commanded to name all of the animals. Bruce also envisions that, in relation to God, humans are invited to explore what He has created in order to glorify Him. Humans are charged to become the steward of what God has made. Bruce also says that some theologians believe that, as a matter of principle, technology can never be and must never be limited—as an expression of the human spirit or of the openness of God's gift of human creativity. However, he argues that scripture, history, and wisdom indicate the need to limit that creativity. He does not believe the notion that just because humans *can* accomplish these wonderful technological feats then they *ought to* carry them out.

What Is a Human Being?

The Biblical view presents the human being as created in *imago dei,* "in the image of God." Individuals are created to have self-awareness of who they are in relation to God. The problems that people have are related to their failed relationship with or disobedience to God. In Genesis, human beings are referred to as "dust" in the sense of being made of the same material as the rest of creation. This might relate today to creation at the molecular level. But the Judeo-Christian tradition views humans as unique—more than just dust or molecules of DNA, but having the spirit and breath of God.

Place of Stewardship

The term *stewardship* is used in the Bible to refer to humans' responsibility for wise and prudent actions in dealing with resources. Thus scientific inquiry, including gene therapy, should be performed responsibly. This also means that people must look at the wider implications and connections to the planet as a whole. Bruce affirms that such a relatively young science as gene therapy and its applications call for use of the "precautionary principle."

IS SOMATIC GENE THERAPY ETHICAL?

Somatic gene therapy, viewed as a medical intervention for helping people, must be undertaken cautiously. Decision makers must consider that there may be greedy, abusive, and exploitive people involved; therefore, regulations are essential to put these in check.

Reverend Demetrios Demopulos, a professor at the Greek Orthodox Cathedral in Brookline, Massachusetts, views the obvious application of the Human Genome Project as the treatment of genetic disorders through gene therapy. Because the target of gene therapy is the somatic cells, he sees few ethical concerns. He believes that treating conditions like sickle cell disease (SCD) and others is consistent with orthodox Christian understanding of appropriate medical treatment. Gene therapy is ethically unacceptable if it goes beyond treatment of disease and is directed at enhancing human performance and making cosmetic changes.

Several religious leaders, including prominent African-American church leaders, contributed to the 2001 issue of *Science* that reported on successful gene therapy experiments for SCD in mice. The group agreed that most religious leaders believe the aim of eliminating suffering coincides with the objectives of medicine and the Christian doctrine of compassion and care.

Is Germ-Line Gene Therapy Acceptable?

The technical problems underlying both embryo and germ-line gene therapy still render it far from feasible. Most Christian thinkers agree that this idea of perfect people or perfecting cosmetic or behavioral traits constitutes a slide down the slippery slope. After all, what is meant by *ideal?* The vision of the perfect body or the ideal shape for humans has changed throughout cultural history. Donald Bruce emphasizes the danger of accepting the ancient Greek concept of the ideal or perfect body, which has no part in the Christian view. He believes that Christians must instead rejoice in diversity and in expanding the notion of the person who is Christ-like.

Islamic Approaches

Gene therapy is one of the modern issues approved by Muslim jurists, as long as it is conducted in accordance with the objectives of Shari'ah and holy Muslim scriptures. According to Dr. Ali Muvy Ed-Deen Al-Qara Daaghi (on IslamOnline.net), certain rules govern therapy in general and gene therapy in particular. The ruling about gene therapy takes into consideration the nature of gene therapy. There is nothing wrong with the procedure as long as no harm is incurred. The Islamic Fiqh Academy, a subsidiary of the Organization of the Islamic Conference that is affiliated with the World Muslim League, addressed this issue at its fifteenth session in 1998. The academy agreed that making the best use of genetic engineering to help protect against and overcome and alleviate the effects of disease is desired, provided that no greater harm is entailed. It is not permissible to conduct research or tamper with the genes of a human being without evaluating future harm. Genetic engineering to attain evil aims is prohibited.

BUDDHISM

Siddhartha Gautama the Buddha, or teacher, lived in the sixth century BC and taught that one must strive for a state of mind called *nirvana*. Nirvana is not a specific set of beliefs, but a state in which one transcends reality and suffering. Unlike the followers of many other religions, Buddhists do not worship a single, omnipresent, all-knowing god, but rather seek to attain the transcendent state through meditation. Rather than being worship-centered, modern Buddhists are action-centered and practice a regimen of simplicity, self-control, and humility.

Buddhists believe in respect for all sentient life, which is defined as beings with a nervous system that have awareness of pain. Important corollaries are the alleviation of suffering and the notion of selfless compassion. Ron Epstein, a professor of Buddhist Studies at the University of California at Berkeley, writes that Buddhist thinkers see problems in genetic engineering that are no different from moral problems experienced elsewhere in daily life: desire, anger, and ignorance. He fears the slippery slope and degree of damage to the environment and to humanity. However, Buddhist thinkers have not been major players in the gene therapy debate, and individuals from countries where Buddhist traditions are strong, such as South Korea and Singapore, are leaders in genetic research, in which their governments are heavily invested.

JUDAISM

According to Dr. Fred Rosner, Director of Mount Sinai Hospital in New York City, applications of genetic engineering such as genetic screening and gene therapy are permissible when used for treatment, cure, or prevention of disease. These types of genetic manipulation do not violate God's natural law but are part of the Biblical mandate to heal. Many genetic diseases, such as Tay-Sachs, are prevalent in Jewish populations. Premarital screening is advised for the purpose of discouraging marriages that risk the perpetuation of a fatal illness. Prenatal screening with the specific intent of aborting an affected fetus is not allowed according to most rabbinical authorities, although a minority view permits the procedure "for great need." Gene manipulation in order to alter such physical characteristics as hair color or facial features is frowned on by Judaism if it serves no medical or psychological purpose.

Jewish believers have three ethical concerns:

- Issues related to education and counseling
- Problems with confidentiality
- Issues of justice

These issues are generally the same as in other bioethical situations that involve newly developed technologies.

HINDUISM

The traditions and beliefs of Hinduism are complex and conflicting at times. In Hindu beliefs, medicine comes to humans as divine knowledge and must conform to the divine will. The Upanishads, the sacred texts, discuss reincarnation and karma, the belief that all actions produce consequences for the future.

According to S. Cromwell Crawford, ThD, University of Hawaii, non-Western sources can contribute to the ethical issues relating to altering human nature. Hindu bioethics comes from three basic principles:

- The transcendent character of human life, expressed in the sanctity and quality of life
- The duty to preserve and guard individual and communal health
- The duty to rectify imbalances in the processes of nature that jeopardize the life and well-being of humans and all other sentient beings

Hindu bioethics does not condemn genetic enhancement as evil, or consider that it meddles with nature or "plays God." Instead, the Hindu belief is that one starts with the whole person, which then permits an evaluation of genetic enhancement by measuring how it can make the person or the person's children better.

The universal principle of *ahimsa* dictates the Hindu outlook. This principle is to do no harm. In a situation in which disease threatens life, the risk of harm may justify genetic treatment. If gene therapy is aimed not at treatment of a serious disease but at nonessential enhancement, *ahimsa* would not support the procedure. Here, the risks would outweigh the benefits. Because health is part of spiritual well-being, efforts at the genetic enhancement of human beings must help, not hinder, the process. Gandhi captured the spirit in these words: "As human beings, our greatness lies not so much in being able to remake the world as in being able to remake ourselves."

Although social and religious questions about gene therapy exist, most people believe that gene therapy to help relieve or alleviate serious and untreatable illnesses is a viable concept. However, genetic enhancement for cosmetic and behavioral changes is not accepted. Most of the arguments against genetic manipulation fall in line with the image of the slippery slope—once it is started, humans do not know what will happen and where it will lead. See Chapter 13, The Future of Gene Therapy, in which hopes for both healing and caution are expressed.

The Future of Gene Therapy

When soldiers in ancient times slashed and cut the enemy, exposing the glistening white bone, some ingenious physician found a unique way to close the wound. While one person held the wound together, another would apply ants or termites. They then pinched off the body of the insect, leaving the strong jaws to hold the wound together. This medical procedure was indeed crude, but sometime in the future, a doctor may think that a surgeon's slashing of cells during an operation is primitive and bizarre. They may think that drugs in current use, with their poisonous side effects, operate in a hit-or-miss manner. Future physicians may rate today's drugs and surgery as harsh treatment; like Hippocrates, they may seek kinder and gentler forms of medical therapy.

Real revolutions in medicine occur only occasionally, and not without resistance and research. The first medical revolution came when scientists recognized that a clean water supply and effective treatment of sewage could lessen the scourge of deadly disease. The second medical revolution was invasive surgery with anesthesia, which allowed physicians to remove a tumor without causing tremendous pain. The third medical revolution was the introduction of antibiotics. The advent of human gene therapy began the fourth revolution in medicine. For gene therapy, the proof of principle exists. In the future, technology must advance to the point of correcting disease at the DNA level.

Although chemical-based drugs have been used successfully for some conditions, for many others there is no treatment, or the available drugs are harsh and have serious, toxic side effects. Medicine is moving rapidly toward therapies that are targeted and based on biology. Gene therapy is on the leading edge of this revolution. In spite of setbacks, gene therapy trials are progressing, as shown in Table 13-1.

This chapter considers some of the challenges that must be met to bring on the genetic revolution and discusses some of the cutting-edge research, including nanomedicine, that may be the wave of the future.

**Table 13-1   Number of Gene Therapy Trials Approved Worldwide,
                     1985–2006**

Year	Number of Trials Approved
1989	1
1990	2
1991	8
1992	14
1993	37
1944	38
1995	67
1996	51
1997	82
1998	68
1999	116
2000	94
2001	107
2002	88
2003	81
2004	91
2005	94
2006 (through July)	28

Adapted by Evelyn B. Kelly from *The Journal of Gene Medicine,* updated July 2006.

In the January 2006 issue of *BioProcess International,* readers were asked the question, how far away are we from safe and efficient gene therapy? Readers responded as follows:

- 12.5 percent thought it would be in 5 years (in 2011)
- 52.5 percent thought it would be in 10 years (in 2016)
- 35.0 percent though it would be in 20 years or more (in 2026)

A summary follows of the comments of these readers, who are scientists involved in research and development:

- Misconduct and inappropriate clinical trials have led to a timeframe that is too long; scientists share responsibility for this.
- There are too many limitations to overcome; additional difficulties will arise when technology develops even more.
- Gene therapy must consider the potential effects on children and grandchildren.
- We do not know what the future will bring; problems may arise 10 to 20 years later for those who are treated today.
- Recent events have created problems for investigators.
- Human bodies were not created for this type of repair.

From this nonscientific survey, one can see the range of ambivalent feelings about gene therapy.

Gene therapy suffered some early setbacks that involved toxic effects and poor success rates. However, Boro Dropulic (2006), CEO of the Lentingen Corporation, alludes to reports by business analysts Frost & Sullivan indicating that the gene therapy market in 2006 reached approximately $125 million and could surpass $6.5 billion by 2011. Technological advances in the design, development, and production of viral vectors are spurring development in gene therapy.

CHALLENGES OF GENE THERAPY

Although gene therapy is not a new field and although dedicated researchers around the world are actively engaged, treatment has seen only limited success. Gene therapy presents one of the greatest technical challenges in all of medicine: introduction of new genes into the cells of the body. Several reasons for the difficulties are reviewed here:

- Gene therapy will work only if several million cells are introduced into the tissue.
- The target must be the correct group of cells in the correct tissue.
- The gene must not incorporate into the wrong cells where a safety hazard would result.
- When the gene reaches its destination, it must be activated to produce the correct protein.
- Vectors—the delivery system—must be able to escape the body's immune system.
- The effect must be lasting; a gene must integrate into the host's genome without disrupting any other gene.

Dr. David M. Bodine, PhD, a senior investigator with the National Genome Research Institute and a member of the American Society of Gene Therapy (ASGT) Advisory Board, spoke on the future of gene therapy with Dr. Melinda Tanzola of Medscape on 7 July 2005. Bodine touts the importance of an organization such as ASGT in bringing together groups who are interested in gene transfer—and ultimately, in gene therapy. The ASGT is composed of many specialists, including biochemists, neurobiologists, oncologists, virologists, and other professionals. The mission of the group is to bring people together and to educate the public.

Dr. Bodine is also pleased that the association is constantly aware of the safety of the various vector systems for delivering gene therapy. He cited the SCID-X experiment in which one child suffered an SAE. However, he believes that more good than bad came of that study.

On the horizon, he expects to see that new tools—genomics, RNAi, chromosomal insulators, and others—will appear in the toolbox for treating disease. Several proof-of-principle treatments have been established, such as those for HD. The problem is to move the success and progress of gene therapy up to the next level. Bodine states that scientists have learned much from the initial tries in the clinic in the past 10 years. Now is the time to go back and study what has been learned and what problems arose. In the second stage, which may arrive around 2010, there will be many clinical trials and new hope for gene therapy.

PROOF OF PRINCIPLE

Scientists use the term *proof of principle* to describe a treatment or procedure that works consistently in preclinical and other settings. For example, studies have shown that SCID patients can benefit from gene therapy. Two examples strongly support the proof of principle:

- Mutations in the gene encoding for the gamma-c cytosine receptor subunit that causes ADA-SCID-X1
- Mutations in the gene for ADA that causes ADA-SCID

Gene therapy has corrected both of these conditions. Some 20 patients are now alive as a direct result of genetic intervention. From these successes, investigators must learn what was done correctly and determine from the failures what went wrong. Thus, gene therapy will become safe and effective enough to become a routine component of medical treatment.

In *The Scientist* (2006), Alain Fischer and Marina Cavazzana-Calvo described in detail their treatment of patients with SCID-X1 and the improvements that can be made to the procedures. Following are their seven steps to better therapy:

1. Amplify target cells for better efficiency. The bone marrow was harvested from the SCID-X1 patient, and CD34+ (a type of cytosine cells) were purified. Finding a way to increase target cells would help in the procedure.
2. Use lentiviruses for increased safety. Scientists found that, in those children in the unsuccessful trials, the viral *LTR* gene activated a proto-oncogene near the integration site and caused the leukemia response. Finding safer and more effective viral vectors is essential. A team from Geneva has found that a 400-bp deletion in HIV-1-3´ UTR impairs the ability of the lentivirus to activate downstream genes.
3. Use AAV when integration is not required. This is an option worth considering for nonreplicating cells when the genetic material does not require integration. Muscle cells and neurons could be engineered in this way because gene expression would not be required for a long period.
4. Alternatively, use targeted integration. Safe sites that are free of oncogenes are another strategy. Scientists at the University of Oregon in Portland used this strategy to correct hereditary tyrosinemia type 1 in the livers of live mice.
5. Fix the problem in the genome. Most of the procedures have involved adding genes to correct problems; gene repair may be a better answer that would avoid the problems of downstream toxicity.
6. Fix the problem functionally. Procedures such as inhibition of abnormal exon expression and gene silencing RNAi are other therapies that may be used.
7. Use a "suicide gene," wherein the gene destroys itself in the process known as apotosis. A drug-inducible suicide gene may increase safety.

RNA SILENCING OR RNA INTERFERENCE

In Chapters 5 through 8, RNA interference (RNAi) or RNA silencing was often mentioned. RNAi is defined as a mechanism in cells that suppresses the expression of genes that determine cell fate, or what happens to the cell in terms of differentiation and survival. This powerful mechanism is found in all mammalian cells. RNAi uses small RNAs of fewer than 30 nucleotides to suppress expression of genes with complementary sequences. Two strategies can introduce RNAs into the cytoplasm of cells:

1. A drug approach, in which RNAs are sent into the cell
2. A gene therapy approach to express precursor RNAs from viral vectors

Every cell has this RNAi machinery and any gene can be targeted with a good deal of specificity, although the targeting procedure is still imperfect. Three years after RNAi was shown to work in mammalian cells, the first phase I clinical studies targeting the VEGF angiogenic pathway in age-related macular degeneration began. Successful silencing in the lung has been achieved by intranasal or intratracheal administration of siRNAs. Other areas that look promising are the mucosal surface of the vagina, subcutaneous tumors, muscle cells, the eye, and the nervous system. This powerful endogenous pathway is exciting to researchers as they seek to treat human disease.

HUMAN GENOME PROJECT (HGP) 2006

When the genome announcement was made in 2001, some people imagined that it would be only a short time until the progress and information contained would be translated into clinical applications. But science does not work this way. Science historian Thomas Kuhn sees these past years as a period of consolidation and more normal science, which might be expressed as a grinding of gears. Researchers have completed the sequencings of the genome of the worm *Caenorhabditis elegans, Pseudomonas aeruginosa,* the principal microbe involved in lung infections of cystic fibrosis, and other organisms. According to some scientists, the past 5 years have been marking time.

However, others see the past 5 years' progress in genomic tools as bringing science into the clinic sooner. The discovery of microRNAs, the small interfering RNAs and the siRNAs, is a great advancement. Five years ago all scientists had was a string of bases; today investigations in basic science are yielding information about what these bases do, and this information can provide the understanding necessary for gene therapy.

Francis Collins, Director of the National Genome Research Institute at NIH, believes that the sequencing of the genomes of *Homo sapiens* and a wide array of other organisms has emerged into a truly quantitative science. The recently completed map of human genetic variation, or HapMap, offers a powerful engine for the discovery of genetic variants that contribute to the risk of common but complex diseases or influence patient response to drugs. The advancing field of pharmacogenomics and the development of diagnostics and personalized treatment and prevention strategies will shed new light on molecular mechanisms underlying many diseases. Collins envisions the HapMap as the most powerful tool to date for unraveling the genetics of common diseases. The next 5 years' road will not be easy, but it is full of hope.   •

In November 2006 researchers released a new version of the human genetic map that fills in missing information explaining how genes are involved in common diseases. The new research questions the assumption that everyone on earth is 99.9 percent identical in his or her genetic makeup. Instead of showing single variations in human DNA, the map presents differences in duplications of large DNA segments called *copy number variants.* These differences help explain why some people are susceptible to illnesses such as AIDS and others are not. Scientists from more than a dozen centers in many countries identified about 3,000 genes with variation in the number of copies of specific DNA segments. The Human Genome mapped the billions of letters that make the genetic codes; the HapMap took the additional step of looking for single variations, called *single-nucleotide polymorphisms,* that have significance in gene activity, especially in susceptibility to disease.

NANOMEDICINE AND GENE THERAPY

Nanomedicine is the application of nanotechnology, the engineering of tiny machines, to the prevention and treatment of diseases and disorders in the human body. In terms of nanomedicine, the body is viewed from the perspective of an intricate machine filled with active, molecular structures. The human body is an active construction site, building, growing, and healing tissue; it is, in every way, like a molecular machine. The cell's genes use the building materials to build biological structures. The word *nanotechnology* is derived from the Greek root *nano,* meaning "one-billionth." In scientific nomenclature, it is written as 10^{-9}.

In 1959 Richard Feynman gave a speech to the American Physics Society challenging scientists to "think small." His classic address, "There's Plenty of Room at the Bottom," asked the participants to consider the question of what would happen if we could arrange atoms one-by-one the way we want. Later, in 1986, Eric Drexler penned *Engine of Creation: The Coming Era of Nanotechnology,* a futuristic book in which he envisioned how molecular technology could be used to create health, not just tackle disease. This entire book may be read at http://www.foresight.org/EOC.

An example of nanotechnology used in gene therapy is the concept of nanoballs, ultra-tiny balls that may deliver DNA more safely and more efficiently. These mini-vectors may bypass the preferred virus vectors that often cannot be given to the same person because the immune system starts attacking them. An example is the use of viruses to deliver the cystic fibrosis (CF) transmembrane regulator genes to patients with CF. Assem Ziady and colleagues have developed a DNA nanoparticle that consists of a plasmid compacted with polyethelene glycol lysine peptides to deliver a copy of the gene. Recently, they found a way to trace where the gene particles are expressed. They injected the firefly luciferase gene—a reporter gene that produces light in the presence of its substrate, luciferin—into the tracheas of mice and followed this procedure with biolumi-nescent imaging. Thus, they were able to find out where the gene particles were expressed as well as the level and duration of expression.

THE NANOROBOTS ARE COMING

In 1920 Czech writer Karel Capek wrote a play titled *R.U.R.* (Rossum's Univer-sal Robots), a fanciful tale that gave us the term *robot,* a mechanical slave. Looking at cutting-edge science and the future, Robert Freitas, a nanomedicine scientist at Zyvek Corporation in Richardson, Texas, envisions billions of minute, self-assembling, computerized robots swarming to the site of injury and sensing, diag-nosing, and activating therapeutic systems. He emphasizes how nanorobots may hold promise for the engineering of enzymes and creation of cell repair machines. In 2000 President Bill Clinton approved $500 million for the National Nanotechnology Initiative, with several divisions that included research on nanomedicine. The overall program coordination occurs through the NIH Bioengineering Consortium.

A MINI-GUIDE FOR INFORMED PEOPLE

Even among educated people, misinformation about genes, heredity, and gene therapy abounds. People pick up bits and pieces from a sensational article or news item and generalize that a cure is at hand. Most people have magical ideas about cutting-edge science—especially gene therapy. Certain simplistic solutions—such as "If you know where the gene is, just change it"—mean nothing.

Here are some ideas that may lend a general perspective on gene therapy:

1. Emphasize that gene therapy has not conquered any disease. Although there have been successes with a few rare conditions, and some trials show promise, no disease has been completely eradicated by the procedure.
2. Understand that the nature of research is very slow and painstaking. Pre-clinical trials in phases I, II, and III may take years in each stage. Most cur-rent gene therapy trials are preclinical or in phase I. It may take 10 years or more to complete a study.
3. Understand how studies to locate genes are done—studies of twins, quanti-tative loci, and transgenic animals. The genes for diseases are located in this way; behavior is much more complicated. (No one has yet located a "fat gene.")
4. Know the terms and be able to intelligently discuss clinical studies, genes, codons, and proteins.
5. Look for examples of good and bad reporting. Stories have claimed that scientists have located a fat gene, gay gene, smoking gene, and even an "I can't stop eating" gene. Reading the study carefully usually reveals that the scientist has found a certain response in an animal. A good report will always state that the topic needs additional study.
6. Get in touch with the NIH to see what studies are open if you are interested in being part of a clinical trial. The NIH Web site is listed in this book. Be

sure to understand the procedure thoroughly and the meaning of informed consent.

7. Check out the books and Web sites that can lay the foundation for people who are interested in genetics and gene therapy. Several are listed at the end of this book. Be a discerning reader and Web surfer. For medical information, go to official Web sites only.

EDUCATION MUST RESPOND

For today's citizens to be informed health consumers, educators must make sure that students understand basic genetics, cell biology, and human physiology. General science textbooks present little about these subjects or do not present enough background to enable students to understand what is happening on the cutting edge of science. These conditions must change in order to create an educated public that is aware of its surroundings and able to make knowledgeable decisions. No child should be left behind in obtaining a foundation for understanding the future. Only with wisdom and understanding of the issues can society benefit from technology and still preserve humanity.

SECTION THREE

References and Resources

Section One, consisting of Chapters 1 through 8, presents the foundations of science that relate to gene therapy. Section One considers the definitions, technology, and historical development of gene therapy, and examines genetic diseases and disorders in a review organized according to their method of inheritance. Section Two, consisting of Chapters 9 though 13, discusses ethical, regulatory and legal, and religious issues related to gene therapy. This last section provides the reader with annotated references and resources consisting of primary documents that have established the foundation of ethical and legal policy decisions related to gene therapy. It concludes with a legal brief of the case of *Gelsinger v. University of Pennsylvania*.

Annotated Primary Source Documents

OATH WRITTEN BY HIPPOCRATES, CA. 400 BC

Chapter 9 addressed ethics and research in history. The word *ethics* comes from the Greek *ethos,* meaning "character." No document embodies the ethics of the medical profession more than the oath accredited to Hippocrates of Cos, written around 400 BC. Hippocrates lived at a time when treatment of the sick involved superstition and incantations. Sometimes very poisonous and dangerous methods were used. Hippocrates disagreed with this and sought to develop a kinder and gentler way of treating people. He was convinced that no treatment should be harsh or inhumane. The oath seeks to protect the rights of patients and to define the proper relationship between physician and patient, stressing in particular the notion of confidentiality.

Later followers of Hippocrates redefined the medical profession in terms of the Hippocratic Oath. During the Dark Ages (i.e., the medieval period) the oath was forgotten but it was revived during the Renaissance and was published around 1525. British physician Thomas Percival first recommended a code of ethics for physicians in 1794.

The Principles of Medical Ethics of the American Medical Association, adopted in 1847 and regularly updated since, similarly state guidelines for physicians. Graduates of medical schools today take the Hippocratic Oath as they begin their practice of medicine. Francis Adams translated the version of the Oath that follows.

Text of the Oath of Hippocrates

I swear by Apollo the physician, and Aesculapius, and Health, and All-heal, and all the gods and goddesses, that, according to my ability and judgment, I will keep this Oath and this stipulation—to reckon him who taught me this Art equally dear to me as my parents, to share my substance with him, and relieve his necessities if required; to look upon his offspring in the same footing as my own brothers, and to teach them this art, if they shall wish to learn it, without fee or stipulation; and that by precept, lecture, and every other mode of instruction, I will impart a knowledge of the Art to my own sons, and those of my teachers, and to disciples bound by a stipulation and oath according to the law of medicine, but to none others. I will follow that system of regimen which, according to my ability and judgment, I consider for the benefit of my patients, and abstain from whatever is deleterious and mischievous. I will give no deadly medicine to any one if asked, nor suggest any such counsel; and in like manner I will not give to a woman a pessary to produce abortion. With purity and with holiness I will pass my life and practice my Art. I will not cut persons laboring under the stone, but will leave this to be done by men who are practitioners of this work. Into whatever houses I enter, I will go into them for the benefit of the sick, and will abstain from every voluntary act of mischief and corruption; and further from the seduction of females or males, of freemen and slaves. Whatever, in connection with my professional practice or not, in connection with it, I see or hear, in the life of men, which ought not to be spoken of abroad, I will not divulge, as reckoning that all such should be kept secret. While I continue to keep this Oath unviolated, may it be granted to me to enjoy life and the practice of the art, respected by all men, in all times! But should I trespass and violate this Oath, may the reverse be my lot!

THE BERLIN CODE OF 1900

As scientific information expanded at the end of the nineteenth century, many investigators began to ponder ethical questions about certain experiments conducted using human subjects. Rudolf Virchow, a microbiologist in Berlin, Germany, had serious reservations about some of the trials undertaken in the name of science. When bacteriologist and physician Albert Ludwig Neisser isolated the spirochete organism believed to cause syphilis, he inoculated some unsuspecting subjects with serum from patients with the disease. Virchow was outraged by this lack of concern for human begins, and he convinced the Berlin City Council to adopt a code of conduct.

This code was one of the first and strongest codes to specify ethical considerations to be observed in conducting medical research. The Code was short-lived, however, and in 1931 Adolph Hitler signed a memo stating that it would not apply to Jews, gypsies, people with mental disabilities, and others. He said these people were not citizens and not entitled to the protection of the Code. However, the Berlin Code remains an important historical document for having made a powerful statement. It can be accessed at http://www.geocities.com/artandersonmd/00prussion1900.jpg.

Text of the Berlin Code

The Royal Prussian Minister of Religious, Educational and Medical Affairs
      Directive to all medical directors of university hospitals, polyclinics,
and other hospitals

  I.   I advise the medical directors of university hospitals, polyclinics, and all
other hospitals that all medical interventions for other than diagnostic,
healing, and immunization purposes, regardless of other legal or moral
authorization, are excluded under all circumstances, if
      (1) the human subject is a minor or not competent due to other reasons;
      (2) the human subject has not given his unambiguous consent;
      (3) the consent is not preceded by a proper explanation of the possible neg-
ative consequences of the intervention.
 II. At the same time I determine that
      (1) interventions of this kind are to be only performed by the medical
director himself or with his special authorization;
      (2) in all cases of these interventions the fulfillment of the requirements of
I (1–3) and II (1), as well as all further circumstances of the case, are
documented in the medical record.
III. The existing instructions about medical interventions for diagnostic, healing, and immunization purposes are not affected by these instructions.

Berlin, 29 December 1900
The Minister for Religious ec. Affairs
Studt

THE NUREMBERG CODE

The Nuremberg Code was created after World War II in response to medical
abuses by some physicians in Hitler's Germany. The Code was written after the trials
in Nuremberg, Germany, in 1946. The object of concern is medical experiments
and research. The Code demands the voluntary informed consent of subjects;
requires that experiments on human subjects be based on the results of animal
experimentation; demands that all mental and physical suffering be eliminated; and
prohibits any experiments that might result in death or prolonged illness.

The Nuremberg Military Tribunal's decision in the case of *United States v.
Karl Brandt et al.* includes what is now called the Nuremberg Code, a ten-point
statement delimiting permissible medical experimentation on human subjects.
According to this statement, human experimentation is justified only if its results

"Permissible Medical Experiments." Trials of War Criminals before the Nuremberg Military
Tribunals under Control Council Law No. 10: Nuremberg, October 1946–April 1949. Washington:
U.S. Government Printing Office (n.d.), vol. 2, pp. 181–2.

benefit society and it is carried out in accord with basic principles that "satisfy moral, ethical, and legal concepts." To some extent, the Nuremberg Code has been superseded by the Declaration of Helsinki as a guide for human experimentation because the Code fails to address Clinical Research in Patients with Illnesses.

Text of the Nuremberg Code

1. The voluntary consent of the human subject is absolutely essential.
This means that the person involved should have legal capacity to give consent; should be so situated as to be able to exercise free power of choice, without the intervention of any element of force, fraud, deceit, duress, overreaching, or other ulterior form of constraint or coercion; and should have sufficient knowledge and comprehension of the elements of the subject matter involved as to enable him to make an understanding and enlightened decision. This latter element requires that before the acceptance of an affirmative decision by the experimental subject there should be made known to him the nature, duration, and purpose of the experiment; the method and means by which it is to be conducted; all inconveniences and hazards reasonably to be expected; and the effects upon his health or person which may possibly come from his participation in the experiment.

The duty and responsibility for ascertaining the quality of the consent rests upon each individual who initiates, directs or engages in the experiment. It is a personal duty and responsibility which may not be delegated to another with impunity.

2. The experiment should be such as to yield fruitful results for the good of society, unprocurable by other methods or means of study, and not random and unnecessary in nature.

3. The experiment should be so designed and based on the results of animal experimentation and a knowledge of the natural history of the disease or other problem under study that the anticipated results will justify the performance of the experiment.

4. The experiment should be so conducted as to avoid all unnecessary physical and mental suffering and injury.

5. No experiment should be conducted where there is an a priori reason to believe that death or disabling injury will occur; except, perhaps, in those experiments where the experimental physicians also serve as subjects.

6. The degree of risk to be taken should never exceed that determined by the humanitarian importance of the problem to be solved by the experiment.

7. Proper preparations should be made and adequate facilities provided to protect the experimental subject against even remote possibilities of injury, disability, or death.

8. The experiment should be conducted only by scientifically qualified persons. The highest degree of skill and care should be required through all stages of the experiment of those who conduct or engage in the experiment.

9. During the course of the experiment the human subject should be at liberty to bring the experiment to an end if he has reached the physical or mental state where continuation of the experiment seems to him to be impossible.

10. During the course of the experiment the scientist in charge must be prepared to terminate the experiment at any stage, if he has probable cause to believe, in the exercise of the good faith, superior skill and careful judgment required of him that a continuation of the experiment is likely to result in injury, disability, or death to the experimental subject.

THE DECLARATION OF HELSINKI

The Declaration of Helsinki provides detailed guidelines for biomedical research involving humans, and serves as an update of the Nuremberg Code. It was established during the decade between 1964 and 1974. It sets forth principles for those involved in experimentation, and provides guidance in ethical behavior for those conducting clinical and nonclinical biomedical research.

Text of the Declaration of Helsinki

WORLD MEDICAL ASSOCIATION [WMA] DECLARATION OF HELSINKI

Ethical Principles for Medical Research Involving Human Subjects

1. The World Medical Association has developed the Declaration of Helsinki as a statement of ethical principles to provide guidance to physicians and other participants in medical research involving human subjects. Medical research involving human subjects includes research on identifiable human material or identifiable data.

2. It is the duty of the physician to promote and safeguard the health of the people. The physician's knowledge and conscience are dedicated to the fulfillment of this duty.

The Declaration of Helsinki is an official policy document of the World Medical Association, the global representative body for physicians. Adopted by the WMA General Assembly in Helsinki, Finland, June 1964, and amended by the 29th WMA General Assembly in Tokyo, Japan, October 1975; by the 35th WMA General Assembly in Venice, Italy, October 1983; by the 41st WMA General Assembly in Hong Kong, September 1989; by the 48th MWA General Assembly in Somerset-West, Republic of South Africa, October 1996; and by the 52nd WMA General Assembly in Edinburgh, Scotland, October 2000. Note of clarification on Paragraph 29 was added by the WMA General Assembly in Washington, 2002. Note of clarification on Paragraph 30 was added by the WMA General Assembly in Tokyo, 2004.

3. The Declaration of Geneva of the World Medical Association binds the physician with the words, "The health of my patient will be my first consideration," and the International Code of Medical Ethics declares that "A physician shall act only in the patient's interest when providing medical care which might have the effect of weakening the physical and mental condition of the patient."

4. Medical progress is based on research which ultimately must rest in part on experimentation involving human subjects.

5. In medical research on human subjects, considerations related to the well-being of the human subject should take precedence over the interests of science and society.

6. The primary purpose of medical research involving human subjects is to improve prophylactic, diagnostic and therapeutic procedures and the understanding of the aetiology and pathogenesis of disease. Even the best proven prophylactic, diagnostic, and therapeutic methods must continuously be challenged through research for their effectiveness, efficiency, accessibility and quality.

7. In current medical practice and in medical research, most prophylactic, diagnostic and therapeutic procedures involve risks and burdens.

8. Medical research is subject to ethical standards that promote respect for all human beings and protect their health and rights. Some research populations are vulnerable and need special protection. The particular needs of the economically and medically disadvantaged must be recognized. Special attention is also required for those who cannot give or refuse consent for themselves, for those who may be subject to giving consent under duress, for those who will not benefit personally from the research and for those for whom the research is combined with care.

9. Research Investigators should be aware of the ethical, legal and regulatory requirements for research on human subjects in their own countries as well as applicable international requirements. No national ethical, legal or regulatory requirement should be allowed to reduce or eliminate any of the protections for human subjects set forth in this Declaration.

Basic Principles for All Medical Research

10. It is the duty of the physician in medical research to protect the life, health, privacy, and dignity of the human subject.

11. Medical research involving human subjects must conform to generally accepted scientific principles, be based on a thorough knowledge of the scientific literature, other relevant sources of information, and on adequate laboratory and, where appropriate, animal experimentation.

12. Appropriate caution must be exercised in the conduct of research which may affect the environment, and the welfare of animals used for research must be respected.

13. The design and performance of each experimental procedure involving human subjects should be clearly formulated in an experimental protocol. This protocol should be submitted for consideration, comment, guidance, and where appropriate, approval to a specially appointed ethical review committee, which must be independent of the investigator, the sponsor or any other kind of undue influence. This independent committee should be in conformity with the laws and regulations of the country in which the research experiment is performed. The committee has the right to monitor ongoing trials. The researcher has the obligation to provide monitoring information to the committee, especially any serious adverse events. The researcher should also submit to the committee, for review, information regarding funding, sponsors, institutional affiliations, other potential conflicts of interest and incentives for subjects.

14. The research protocol should always contain a statement of the ethical considerations involved and should indicate that there is compliance with the principles enunciated in this Declaration.

15. Medical research involving human subjects should be conducted only by scientifically qualified persons and under the supervision of a clinically competent medical person. The responsibility for the human subject must always rest with a medically qualified person and never rest on the subject of the research, even though the subject has given consent.

16. Every medical research project involving human subjects should be preceded by careful assessment of predictable risks and burdens in comparison with foreseeable benefits to the subject or to others. This does not preclude the participation of healthy volunteers in medical research. The design of all studies should be publicly available.

17. Physicians should abstain from engaging in research projects involving human subjects unless they are confident that the risks involved have been adequately assessed and can be satisfactorily managed. Physicians should cease any investigation if the risks are found to outweigh the potential benefits or if there is conclusive proof of positive and beneficial results.

18. Medical research involving human subjects should only be conducted if the importance of the objective outweighs the inherent risks and burdens to the subject. This is especially important when the human subjects are healthy volunteers.

19. Medical research is only justified if there is a reasonable likelihood that the populations in which the research is carried out stand to benefit from the results of the research.

20. The subjects must be volunteers and informed participants in the research project.

21. The right of research subjects to safeguard their integrity must always be respected. Every precaution should be taken to respect the privacy of the subject, the confidentiality of the patient's information and to minimize the impact of the study on the subject's physical and mental integrity and on the personality of the subject.

22. In any research on human beings, each potential subject must be adequately informed of the aims, methods, sources of funding, any possible conflicts of interest, institutional affiliations of the researcher, the anticipated benefits and potential risks of the study and the discomfort it may entail. The subject should be informed of the right to abstain from participation in the study or to withdraw consent to participate at any time without reprisal. After ensuring that the subject has understood the information, the physician should then obtain the subject's freely-given informed consent, preferably in writing. If the consent cannot be obtained in writing, the non-written consent must be formally documented and witnessed.

23. When obtaining informed consent for the research project the physician should be particularly cautious if the subject is in a dependent relationship with the physician or may consent under duress. In that case the informed consent should be obtained by a well-informed physician who is not engaged in the investigation and who is completely independent of this relationship.

24. For a research subject who is legally incompetent, physically or mentally incapable of giving consent or is a legally incompetent minor, the investigator must obtain informed consent from the legally authorized representative in accordance with applicable law. These groups should not be included in research unless the research is necessary to promote the health of the population represented and this research cannot instead be performed on legally competent persons.

25. When a subject deemed legally incompetent, such as a minor child, is able to give assent to decisions about participation in research, the investigator must obtain that assent in addition to the consent of the legally authorized representative.

26. Research on individuals from whom it is not possible to obtain consent, including proxy or advance consent, should be done only if the physical/mental condition that prevents obtaining informed consent is a necessary characteristic of the research population. The specific reasons for involving research subjects with a condition that renders them unable to give informed consent should be stated in the experimental protocol for consideration and approval of the review committee.

27. The protocol should state that consent to remain in the research should be obtained as soon as possible from the individual or a legally authorized surrogate.

28. Both authors and publishers have ethical obligations. In publication of the results of research, the investigators are obliged to preserve the accuracy of the results. Negative as well as positive results should be published or otherwise publicly available. Sources of funding, institutional affiliations and any possible conflicts of interest should be declared in the publication. Reports of experimentation not in accordance with the principles laid down in this Declaration should not be accepted for publication.

Additional Principles for Medical Research
Combined with Medical Care

29.   The physician may combine medical research with medical care, only to the extent that the research is justified by its potential prophylactic, diagnostic or therapeutic value. When medical research is combined with medical care, additional standards apply to protect the patients who are research subjects. The benefits, risks, burdens and effectiveness of a new method should be tested against those of the best current prophylactic, diagnostic, and therapeutic methods. This does not exclude the use of placebo, or no treatment, in studies where no proven prophylactic, diagnostic or therapeutic method exists. [See Note of Clarification.]

30.   At the conclusion of the study, every patient entered into the study should be assured of access to the best proven prophylactic, diagnostic and therapeutic methods identified by the study. [See Note of Clarification.] The physician should fully inform the patient which aspects of the care are related to the research. The refusal of a patient to participate in a study must never interfere with the patient-physician relationship. In the treatment of a patient, where proven prophylactic, diagnostic and therapeutic methods do not exist or have been ineffective, the physician, with informed consent from the patient, must be free to use unproven or new prophylactic, diagnostic and therapeutic measures, if in the physician's judgement it offers hope of saving life, re-establishing health or alleviating suffering. Where possible, these measures should be made the object of research, designed to evaluate their safety and efficacy. In all cases, new information should be recorded and, where appropriate, published. The other relevant guidelines of this Declaration should be followed.

Note of Clarification to Paragraph 29 of the
WMA Declaration of Helsinki

The WMA hereby reaffirms its position that extreme care must be taken in making use of a placebo-controlled trial and that in general this methodology should only be used in the absence of existing proven therapy. However, a placebo-controlled trial may be ethically acceptable, even if proven therapy is available, under the following circumstances:

- Where for compelling and scientifically sound methodological reasons its use is necessary to determine the efficacy or safety of a prophylactic, diagnostic or therapeutic method; or

- Where a prophylactic, diagnostic or therapeutic method is being investigated for a minor condition and the patients who receive placebo will not be subject to any additional risk of serious or irreversible harm.

All other provisions of the Declaration of Helsinki must be adhered to, especially the need for appropriate ethical and scientific review.

Note of Clarification to Paragraph 30 of the WMA Declaration of Helsinki

The WMA hereby reaffirms its position that it is necessary during the study planning process to identify post-trial access by study participants to prophylactic, diagnostic and therapeutic procedures identified as beneficial in the study or access to other appropriate care. Post-trial access arrangements or other care must be described in the study protocol so the ethical review committee may consider such arrangements during its review.

THE BELMONT REPORT

When the U.S. Public Health Service Syphilis Study revealed that a study of syphilis in Tuskegee, Alabama, had been sanctioned from 1932 to 1972, the world was shocked. That the Service withheld known treatment that could have cured the men who were subjects in the study marked a low point for medical experimentation. These revelations led to the National Research Act (P.L. 93-348) in July 1974, which added restrictions and oversight requirements for research involving human subjects. On 12 July 12 1975, a commission was formed to identify basic ethical principles that should govern any research involving human subjects. The following report is named for the Belmont Conference Center at the Smithsonian Institution.

Text of the Belmont Report

Ethical Principles and Guidelines for the Protection of Human Subjects of Research

---

The National Commission for the Protection of Human Subjects of Biomedical and Behavioral Research

April 18, 1979

AGENCY: Department of Health, Education, and Welfare.

ACTION: Notice of Report for Public Comment.

SUMMARY: On July 12, 1974, the National Research Act (Pub. L. 93-348) was signed into law, thereby creating the National Commission for the Protection of Human Subjects of Biomedical and Behavioral Research. One of the charges to the Commission was to identify the basic ethical principles that should underlie the conduct of biomedical and behavioral research involving human subjects and to develop guidelines which should be followed to assure that such research is conducted in accordance with those principles. In carrying out the above, the Commission was directed to consider: (i) the boundaries between biomedical and behavioral research and the accepted and routine practice of medicine, (ii) the role of assessment of risk-benefit criteria in the determination of the appropriateness of research involving human subjects, (iii) appropriate guidelines for the selection of human subjects for participation in such research, and (iv) the nature and definition of informed consent in various research settings.

The Belmont Report attempts to summarize the basic ethical principles identified by the Commission in the course of its deliberations. It is the outgrowth of an intensive four-day period of discussions that were held in February 1976 at the Smithsonian Institution's Belmont Conference Center supplemented by the monthly deliberations of the Commission that were held over a period of nearly four years. It is a statement of basic ethical principles and guidelines that should assist in resolving the ethical problems that surround the conduct of research with human subjects. By publishing the Report in the Federal Register, and providing reprints upon request, the Secretary intends that it may be made readily available to scientists, members of Institutional Review Boards, and Federal employees. The two-volume Appendix, containing the lengthy reports of experts and specialists who assisted the Commission in fulfilling this part of its charge, is available as DHEW Publication No. (OS) 78-0013 and No. (OS) 78-0014, for sale by the Superintendent of Documents, U.S. Government Printing Office, Washington, D.C. 20402.

Unlike most other reports of the Commission, the Belmont Report does not make specific recommendations for administrative action by the Secretary of Health, Education, and Welfare. Rather, the Commission recommended that the Belmont Report be adopted in its entirety, as a statement of the Department's policy. The Department requests public comment on this recommendation.

ETHICAL PRINCIPLES AND GUIDELINES FOR RESEARCH INVOLVING HUMAN SUBJECTS

Scientific research has produced substantial social benefits. It has also posed some troubling ethical questions. Public attention was drawn to these questions by reported abuses of human subjects in biomedical experiments, especially during the Second World War. During the Nuremberg War Crime Trials, the Nuremberg code was drafted as a set of standards for judging physicians and scientists who had conducted biomedical experiments on concentration camp prisoners. This code became the prototype of many later codes[1] intended to assure that research involving human subjects would be carried out in an ethical manner.

The codes consist of rules—some general, others specific—that guide the investigators or the reviewers of research in their work. Such rules often are inadequate to cover complex situations; at times they come into conflict, and they are frequently difficult to interpret or apply. Broader ethical principles will provide a basis on which specific rules may be formulated, criticized and interpreted.

Three principles, or general prescriptive judgments, that are relevant to research involving human subjects are identified in this statement. Other principles may also be relevant. These three are comprehensive, however, and are stated at a level of generalization that should assist scientists, subjects, reviewers and interested citizens to understand the ethical issues inherent in research involving human subjects. These principles cannot always be applied so as to resolve beyond dispute particular ethical problems. The objective is to provide an analytical framework that will guide the resolution of ethical problems arising from research involving human subjects.

This statement consists of a distinction between research and practice, a discussion of the three basic ethical principles, and remarks about the application of these principles.

Part A. Boundaries between Practice and Research

It is important to distinguish between biomedical and behavioral research, on the one hand, and the practice of accepted therapy on the other, in order to know what activities ought to undergo review for the protection of human subjects of research. The distinction between research and practice is blurred partly because both often occur together (as in research designed to evaluate a therapy) and partly because notable departures from standard practice are often called "experimental" when the terms "experimental" and "research" are not carefully defined.

For the most part, the term "practice" refers to interventions that are designed solely to enhance the well-being of an individual patient or client and that have a reasonable expectation of success. The purpose of medical or behavioral practice is to provide diagnosis, preventive treatment or therapy to particular individuals.[2] By contrast, the term "research" designates an activity designed to test an hypothesis, permit conclusions to be drawn, and thereby to develop or contribute to generalizable knowledge (expressed, for example, in theories, principles, and statements of relationships). Research is usually described in a formal protocol that sets forth an objective and a set of procedures designed to reach that objective.

When a clinician departs in a significant way from standard or accepted practice, the innovation does not, in and of itself, constitute research. The fact that a procedure is "experimental," in the sense of new, untested or different, does not automatically place it in the category of research. Radically new procedures of this description should, however, be made the object of formal research at an early stage in order to determine whether they are safe and effective. Thus, it is the responsibility of medical practice committees, for example, to insist that a major innovation be incorporated into a formal research project.[3]

Research and practice may be carried on together when research is designed to evaluate the safety and efficacy of a therapy. This need not cause any confusion regarding whether or not the activity requires review; the general rule is that if there is any element of research in an activity, that activity should undergo review for the protection of human subjects.

Part B. Basic Ethical Principles

The expression "basic ethical principles" refers to those general judgments that serve as a basic justification for the many particular ethical prescriptions and evaluations of human actions. Three basic principles, among those generally accepted in our cultural tradition, are particularly relevant to the ethics of research involving human subjects: the principles of respect for persons, beneficence and justice.

1. Respect for Persons. Respect for persons incorporates at least two ethical convictions: first, that individuals should be treated as autonomous agents; and second, that persons with diminished autonomy are entitled to protection. The principle of respect for persons thus divides into two separate moral requirements: the requirement to acknowledge autonomy and the requirement to protect those with diminished autonomy.

An autonomous person is an individual capable of deliberation about personal goals and of acting under the direction of such deliberation. To respect autonomy is to give weight to autonomous persons' considered opinions and choices while refraining from obstructing their actions unless they are clearly detrimental to others. To show lack of respect for an autonomous agent is to repudiate that person's considered judgments, to deny an individual the freedom to act on those considered judgments, or to withhold information necessary to make a considered judgment, when there are no compelling reasons to do so.

However, not every human being is capable of self-determination. The capacity for self-determination matures during an individual's life, and some individuals lose this capacity wholly or in part because of illness, mental disability, or circumstances that severely restrict liberty. Respect for the immature and the incapacitated may require protecting them as they mature or while they are incapacitated.

Some persons are in need of extensive protection, even to the point of excluding them from activities which may harm them; other persons require little protection beyond making sure they undertake activities freely and with awareness of possible adverse consequence. The extent of protection afforded should depend upon the risk of harm and the likelihood of benefit. The judgment that any individual lacks autonomy should be periodically reevaluated and will vary in different situations.

In most cases of research involving human subjects, respect for persons demands that subjects enter into the research voluntarily and with adequate information. In some situations, however, application of the principle is not obvious. The involvement of prisoners as subjects of research provides an instructive example. On the one hand, it would seem that the principle of respect for persons requires that prisoners not be deprived of the opportunity to volunteer for research. On the other hand, under prison conditions they may be subtly coerced or unduly influenced to engage in research activities for which they would not otherwise volunteer. Respect for persons would then dictate that prisoners be protected. Whether to allow prisoners to "volunteer" or to "protect" them presents a dilemma. Respecting persons, in most hard cases, is often a matter of balancing competing claims urged by the principle of respect itself.

2. Beneficence. Persons are treated in an ethical manner not only by respecting their decisions and protecting them from harm, but also by making efforts to secure their well-being. Such treatment falls under the principle of beneficence. The term "beneficence" is often understood to cover acts of kindness or charity that go beyond strict obligation. In this document, beneficence is understood in a stronger sense, as an obligation. Two general rules have been formulated as complementary expressions of beneficent actions in this sense: (1) do not harm and (2) maximize possible benefits and minimize possible harms.

The Hippocratic "do no harm" maxim has long been a fundamental principle of medical ethics. Claude Bernard extended it to the realm of research, saying that one should not injure one person regardless of the benefits that might come to others. However, even avoiding harm requires learning what is harmful; and, in the process of obtaining this information, persons may be exposed to risk of harm. Further, the Hippocratic Oath requires physicians to benefit their patients "according to their best judgment." Learning what will in fact benefit may require exposing persons to risk. The problem posed by these imperatives is to decide when it is justifiable to seek certain benefits despite the risks involved, and when the benefits should be foregone because of the risks.

The obligations of beneficence affect both individual investigators and society at large, because they extend both to particular research projects and to the entire enterprise of research. In the case of particular projects, investigators and members of their institutions are obliged to give forethought to the maximization of benefits and the reduction of risk that might occur from the research investigation. In the case of scientific research in general, members of the larger society are obliged to recognize the longer term benefits and risks that may result from the improvement of knowledge and from the development of novel medical, psychotherapeutic, and social procedures.

The principle of beneficence often occupies a well-defined justifying role in many areas of research involving human subjects. An example is found in research involving children. Effective ways of treating childhood diseases and fostering healthy development are benefits that serve to justify research involving children—even when individual research subjects are not direct beneficiaries. Research also makes it possible to avoid the harm that may result from the application of previously accepted routine practices that on closer investigation turn out to be dangerous. But the role of the principle of beneficence is not always so unambiguous. A difficult ethical problem remains, for example, about research that presents more than minimal risk without immediate prospect of direct benefit to the children involved. Some have argued that such research is inadmissible, while others have pointed out that this limit would rule out much research promising great benefit to children in the future. Here again, as with all hard cases, the different claims covered by the principle of beneficence may come into conflict and force difficult choices.

3. Justice. Who ought to receive the benefits of research and bear its burdens? This is a question of justice, in the sense of "fairness in distribution" or "what is deserved." An injustice occurs when some benefit to which a person is entitled is denied without good reason or when some burden is imposed unduly. Another way of conceiving the principle of justice is that equals ought to be treated equally. However, this statement requires explication. Who is equal and who is unequal? What considerations justify departure from equal distribution? Almost all commentators allow that distinctions based on experience, age, deprivation, competence, merit and position do sometimes constitute criteria justifying differential treatment for certain purposes. It is necessary, then, to explain in what respects people should be treated equally. There are several widely accepted formulations of just ways to distribute burdens and benefits. Each formulation mentions some relevant property on the basis of which burdens and benefits should be distributed. These formulations are (1) to each person an equal share, (2) to each person according to individual need, (3) to each person according to individual effort, (4) to each person according to societal contribution, and (5) to each person according to merit.

Questions of justice have long been associated with social practices such as punishment, taxation and political representation. Until recently these questions have not generally been associated with scientific research. However, they are foreshadowed even in the earliest reflections on the ethics of research involving human subjects. For example, during the nineteenth and early twentieth centuries the burdens of serving as research subjects fell largely upon poor ward patients, while the benefits of improved medical care flowed primarily to private patients. Subsequently, the exploitation of unwilling prisoners as research subjects in Nazi concentration camps was condemned as a particularly flagrant injustice. In this country, in the 1940s, the Tuskegee syphilis study used disadvantaged, rural black men to study the untreated course of a disease that is by no means confined to that population. These subjects were deprived of demonstrably effective treatment in order not to interrupt the project, long after such treatment became generally available.

Against this historical background, it can be seen how conceptions of justice are relevant to research involving human subjects. For example, the selection of research subjects needs to be scrutinized in order to determine whether some classes (e.g., welfare patients, particular racial and ethnic minorities, or persons confined to institutions) are being systematically selected simply because of their easy availability, their compromised position, or their manipulability, rather than for reasons directly related to the problem being studied. Finally, whenever research supported by public funds leads to the development of therapeutic devices and procedures, justice demands both that these not provide advantages only to those who can afford them and that such research should not unduly involve persons from groups unlikely to be among the beneficiaries of subsequent applications of the research.

Part C. Applications

Applications of the general principles to the conduct of research leads to consideration of the following requirements: informed consent, risk/benefit assessment, and the selection of subjects of research.

1. Informed Consent. Respect for persons requires that subjects, to the degree that they are capable, be given the opportunity to choose what shall or shall not happen to them. This opportunity is provided when adequate standards for informed consent are satisfied.

While the importance of informed consent is unquestioned, controversy prevails over the nature and possibility of an informed consent. Nonetheless, there is widespread agreement that the consent process can be analyzed as containing three elements: information, comprehension and voluntariness.

Information. Most codes of research establish specific items for disclosure intended to assure that subjects are given sufficient information. These items generally include: the research procedure[s]; their purposes, risks and anticipated benefits; alternative procedures (where therapy is involved); and a statement offering the subject the opportunity to ask questions and to withdraw at any time from the research. Additional items have been proposed, including how subjects are selected, the person responsible for the research, etc.

However, a simple listing of items does not answer the question of what the standard should be for judging how much and what sort of information should be provided. One standard frequently invoked in medical practice, namely the information commonly provided by practitioners in the field or in the locale, is inadequate since research takes place precisely when a common understanding does not exist. Another standard, currently popular in malpractice law, requires the practitioner to reveal the information that reasonable persons would wish to know in order to make a decision regarding their care. This, too, seems insufficient since the research subject, being in essence a volunteer, may wish to know considerably more about risks gratuitously undertaken than do patients who deliver themselves into the hand of a clinician for needed care. It may be that a standard of "the reasonable volunteer" should be proposed: the extent and nature of information should be such that persons, knowing that the procedure is neither necessary for their care nor perhaps fully understood, can decide whether they wish to participate in the furthering of knowledge. Even when some direct benefit to them is anticipated, the subjects should understand clearly the range of risk and the voluntary nature of participation.

A special problem of consent arises where informing subjects of some pertinent aspect of the research is likely to impair the validity of the research. In many cases, it is sufficient to indicate to subjects that they are being invited to participate in research of which some features will not be revealed until the research is concluded. In all cases of research involving incomplete disclosure, such research is justified only if it is clear that (1) incomplete disclosure is truly necessary to accomplish the goals of the research, (2) there are no undisclosed risks to subjects that are more than minimal, and (3) there is an adequate plan for debriefing subjects, when appropriate, and for dissemination of research results to them. Information about risks should never be withheld for the purpose of eliciting the cooperation of subjects, and truthful answers should always be given to direct questions about the research. Care should be taken to distinguish cases in which disclosure would destroy or invalidate the research from cases in which disclosure would simply inconvenience the investigator.

Comprehension. The manner and context in which information is conveyed is as important as the information itself. For example, presenting information in a disorganized and rapid fashion, allowing too little time for consideration or curtailing opportunities for questioning, all may adversely affect a subject's ability to make an informed choice.

Because the subject's ability to understand is a function of intelligence, rationality, maturity and language, it is necessary to adapt the presentation of the information to the subject's capacities. Investigators are responsible for ascertaining that the subject has comprehended the information. While there is always an obligation to ascertain that the information about risk to subjects is complete and adequately comprehended, when the risks are more serious, that obligation increases. On occasion, it may be suitable to give some oral or written tests of comprehension.

Special provision may need to be made when comprehension is severely limited— for example, by conditions of immaturity or mental disability. Each class of subjects that one might consider as incompetent (e.g., infants and young children, mentally disabled patients, the terminally ill and the comatose) should be considered on its own terms. Even for these persons, however, respect requires giving them the opportunity to choose to the extent they are able, whether or not to participate in research. The objections of these subjects to involvement should be honored, unless the research entails providing them a therapy unavailable elsewhere. Respect for persons also requires seeking the permission of other parties in order to protect the subjects from harm. Such persons are thus respected both by acknowledging their own wishes and by the use of third parties to protect them from harm.

The third parties chosen should be those who are most likely to understand the incompetent subject's situation and to act in that person's best interest. The person authorized to act on behalf of the subject should be given an opportunity to observe the research as it proceeds in order to be able to withdraw the subject from the research, if such action appears in the subject's best interest.

Voluntariness. An agreement to participate in research constitutes a valid consent only if voluntarily given. This element of informed consent requires conditions free of coercion and undue influence. Coercion occurs when an overt threat of harm is intentionally presented by one person to another in order to obtain compliance. Undue influence, by contrast, occurs through an offer of an excessive, unwarranted, inappropriate or improper reward or other overture in order to obtain compliance. Also, inducements that would ordinarily be acceptable may become undue influences if the subject is especially vulnerable.

Unjustifiable pressures usually occur when persons in positions of authority or commanding influence—especially where possible sanctions are involved—urge a course of action for a subject. A continuum of such influencing factors exists, however, and it is impossible to state precisely where justifiable persuasion ends and undue influence begins. But undue influence would include actions such as manipulating a person's choice through the controlling influence of a close relative and threatening to withdraw health services to which an individual would otherwise be entitled.

2. Assessment of Risks and Benefits. The assessment of risks and benefits requires a careful arrayal of relevant data, including, in some cases, alternative ways of obtaining the benefits sought in the research. Thus, the assessment presents both an opportunity and a responsibility to gather systematic and comprehensive information about proposed research. For the investigator, it is a means to examine whether the proposed research is properly designed. For a review committee, it is a method for determining whether the risks that will be presented to subjects are justified. For prospective subjects, the assessment will assist the determination whether or not to participate.

The Nature and Scope of Risks and Benefits. The requirement that research be justified on the basis of a favorable risk/benefit assessment bears a close relation to the principle of beneficence, just as the moral requirement that informed consent be obtained is derived primarily from the principle of respect for persons. The term "risk" refers to a possibility that harm may occur. However, when expressions such as "small risk" or "high risk" are used, they usually refer (often ambiguously) both to the chance (probability) of experiencing a harm and the severity (magnitude) of the envisioned harm.

The term "benefit" is used in the research context to refer to something of positive value related to health or welfare. Unlike "risk," "benefit" is not a term that expresses probabilities. Risk is properly contrasted to probability of benefits, and benefits are properly contrasted with harms rather than risks of harm. Accordingly, so-called risk/benefit assessments are concerned with the probabilities and magnitudes of possible harm and anticipated benefits. Many kinds of possible harms and benefits need to be taken into account. There are, for example, risks of psychological harm, physical harm, legal harm, social harm and economic harm and the corresponding benefits. While the most likely types of harms to research subjects are those of psychological or physical pain or injury, other possible kinds should not be overlooked.

Risks and benefits of research may affect the individual subjects, the families of the individual subjects, and society at large (or special groups of subjects in society). Previous codes and Federal regulations have required that risks to subjects be outweighed by the sum of both the anticipated benefit to the subject, if any, and the anticipated benefit to society in the form of knowledge to be gained from the research. In balancing these different elements, the risks and benefits affecting the immediate research subject will normally carry special weight. On the other hand, interests other than those of the subject may on some occasions be sufficient by themselves to justify the risks involved in the research, so long as the subjects' rights have been protected. Beneficence thus requires that we protect against risk of harm to subjects and also that we be concerned about the loss of the substantial benefits that might be gained from research.

The Systematic Assessment of Risks and Benefits. It is commonly said that benefits and risks must be "balanced" and shown to be "in a favorable ratio." The metaphorical character of these terms draws attention to the difficulty of making precise judgments. Only on rare occasions will quantitative techniques be available for the scrutiny of research protocols. However, the idea of systematic, nonarbitrary analysis of risks and benefits should be emulated insofar as possible. This ideal requires those making decisions about the justifiability of research to be thorough in the accumulation and assessment of information about all aspects of the research, and to consider alternatives systematically. This procedure renders the assessment of research more rigorous and precise, while making communication between review board members and investigators less subject to misinterpretation, misinformation and conflicting judgments. Thus, there should first be a determination of the validity of the presuppositions of the research; then the nature, probability and magnitude of risk should be distinguished with as much clarity as possible. The method of ascertaining risks should be explicit, especially where there is no alternative to the use of such vague categories as small or slight risk. It should also be determined whether an investigator's estimates of the probability of harm or benefits are reasonable, as judged by known facts or other available studies.

Finally, assessment of the justifiability of research should reflect at least the following considerations: (i) Brutal or inhumane treatment of human subjects is never morally justified. (ii) Risks should be reduced to those necessary to achieve the research objective. It should be determined whether it is in fact necessary to use human subjects at all. Risk can perhaps never be entirely eliminated, but it can often be reduced by careful attention to alternative procedures. (iii) When research involves significant risk of serious impairment, review committees should be extraordinarily insistent on the justification of the risk (looking usually to the likelihood of benefit to the subject—or, in some rare cases, to the manifest voluntariness of the participation). (iv) When vulnerable populations are involved in research, the appropriateness of involving them should itself be demonstrated. A number of variables go into such judgments, including the nature and degree of risk, the condition of the particular population involved, and the nature and level of the anticipated benefits. (v) Relevant risks and benefits must be thoroughly arrayed in documents and procedures used in the informed consent process.

3. Selection of Subjects. Just as the principle of respect for persons finds expression in the requirements for consent, and the principle of beneficence in risk/benefit assessment, the principle of justice gives rise to moral requirements that there be fair procedures and outcomes in the selection of research subjects.

Justice is relevant to the selection of subjects of research at two levels: the social and the individual. Individual justice in the selection of subjects would require that researchers exhibit fairness: thus, they should not offer potentially beneficial research only to some patients who are in their favor or select only "undesirable" persons for risky research. Social justice requires that distinction be drawn between classes of subjects that ought, and ought not, to participate in any particular kind of research, based on the ability of members of that class to bear burdens and on the appropriateness of placing further burdens on already burdened persons. Thus, it can be considered a matter of social justice that there is an order of preference in the selection of classes of subjects (e.g., adults before children) and that some classes of potential subjects (e.g., the institutionalized mentally infirm or prisoners) may be involved as research subjects, if at all, only on certain conditions.

Injustice may appear in the selection of subjects, even if individual subjects are selected fairly by investigators and treated fairly in the course of research. This injustice arises from social, racial, sexual and cultural biases institutionalized in society. Thus, even if individual researchers are treating their research subjects fairly, and even if [institutional review boards] IRBs are taking care to assure that subjects are selected fairly within a particular institution, unjust social patterns may nevertheless appear in the overall distribution of the burdens and benefits of research. Although individual institutions or investigators may not be able to resolve a problem that is pervasive in their social setting, they can consider distributive justice in selecting research subjects.

Some populations, especially institutionalized ones, are already burdened in many ways by their infirmities and environments. When research is proposed that involves risks and does not include a therapeutic component, other less burdened classes of persons should be called upon first to accept these risks of research, except where the research is directly related to the specific conditions of the class involved. Also, even though public funds for research may often flow in the same directions as public funds for health care, it seems unfair that populations dependent on public health care constitute a pool of preferred research subjects if more advantaged populations are likely to be the recipients of the benefits.

One special instance of injustice results from the involvement of vulnerable subjects. Certain groups, such as racial minorities, the economically disadvantaged, the very sick, and the institutionalized may continually be sought as research subjects, owing to their ready availability in settings where research is conducted. Given their dependent status and their frequently compromised capacity for free consent, they should be protected against the danger of being involved in research solely for administrative convenience, or because they are easy to manipulate as a result of their illness or socioeconomic condition.

---

1. Since 1945, various codes for the proper and responsible conduct of human experimentation in medical research have been adopted by different organizations. The best known of these codes are the Nuremberg Code of 1947, the Helsinki Declaration of 1964 (revised in 1975), and the 1971 Guidelines (codified into Federal Regulations in 1974) issued by the U.S. Department of Health, Education, and Welfare. Codes for the conduct of social and behavioral research

have also been adopted, the best known being that of the American Psychological Association, published in 1973.

2. Although practice usually involves interventions designed solely to enhance the well-being of a particular individual, interventions are sometimes applied to one individual for the enhancement of the well-being of another (e.g., blood donation, skin grafts, and organ transplants) or an intervention may have the dual purpose of enhancing the well-being of a particular individual, and, at the same time, providing some benefit to others (e.g., vaccination, which protects both the person who is vaccinated and society generally). The fact that some forms of practice have elements other than immediate benefit to the individual receiving an intervention, however, should not confuse the general distinction between research and practice. Even when a procedure applied in practice may benefit some other person, it remains an intervention designed to enhance the well-being of a particular individual or groups of individuals; thus, it is practice and need not be reviewed as research.

3. Because the problems related to social experimentation may differ substantially from those of biomedical and behavioral research, the Commission specifically declines to make any policy determination regarding such research at this time. Rather, the Commission believes that the problem ought to be addressed by one of its successor bodies.

NIH GUIDELINES FOR DNA RESEARCH

The *National Institutes for Health Guidelines* for research involving recombinant DNA are very complex. Nevertheless, scientists are expected to know and digest every ruling. They must know all the laws and determinations of the *Guidelines.* Not knowing them or not abiding by them can get a research team into great difficulty. Included in this section of Appendix A are only the outline and a few beginning items.

Text of the *NIH Guidelines* for DNA Research

NIH GUIDELINES FOR RESEARCH
INVOLVING RECOMBINANT
DNA MOLECULES
(NIH GUIDELINES)
April 2002
Visit the OBA Web site at
http://www4.od.nih.gov/oba
FOR CURRENT INFORMATION ON GUIDELINES, PROTOCOLS,
PRINCIPAL INVESTIGATORS, MEETINGS, AND INFORMATION
ABOUT UPCOMING GENE THERAPY POLICY CONFERENCES

DEPARTMENT OF HEALTH AND HUMAN SERVICES
NATIONAL INSTITUTES OF HEALTH
GUIDELINES FOR RESEARCH INVOLVING RECOMBINANT DNA
MOLECULES (NIH GUIDELINES)

These *NIH Guidelines* supersede all earlier versions and shall be in effect until further notice.

SECTION I. SCOPE OF THE *NIH GUIDELINES*

Section I-A.   Purpose

The purpose of the *NIH Guidelines* is to specify practices for constructing and handling: (i) recombinant deoxyribonucleic acid (DNA) molecules, and (ii) organisms and viruses containing recombinant DNA molecules.

Section I-A-1. Any recombinant DNA experiment, which according to the *NIH Guidelines* requires approval by NIH, must be submitted to NIH or to another Federal agency that has jurisdiction for review and approval. Once approvals, or other applicable clearances, have been obtained from a Federal agency other than NIH (whether the experiment is referred to that agency by NIH or sent directly there by the submitter), the experiment may proceed without the necessity for NIH review or approval. (See exception in *Section I-A-1-a* regarding requirement for human gene transfer protocol registration.)

Section I-A-1-a. For experiments involving the deliberate transfer of recombinant DNA, or DNA or RNA derived from recombinant DNA, into human research participants (human gene transfer), no research participant shall be enrolled (see definition of enrollment in *Section I-E-7*) until the RAC review process has been completed (see *Appendix M-I-B, RAC Review Requirements*); Institutional Biosafety Committee (IBC) approval (from the clinical trial site) has been obtained; Institutional Review Board approval has been obtained; and all applicable regulatory authorization(s) have been obtained.

For a clinical trial site that is added after the RAC review process, no research participant shall be enrolled (see definition of enrollment in *Section I-E-7*) at the clinical trial site until the following documentation has been submitted to NIH OBA: (1) IBC approval (from the clinical trial site); (2) Institutional Review Board approval; (3) Institutional Review Board-approved informed consent document; and (4) curriculum vitae of the principal investigator(s) (no more than two pages in biographical sketch format); and (5) NIH grant number(s) if applicable.

Section I-B.   Definition of Recombinant DNA Molecules

In the context of the *NIH Guidelines,* recombinant DNA molecules are defined as either: (i) molecules that are constructed outside living cells by joining natural or synthetic DNA segments to DNA molecules that can replicate in a living cell, or (ii) molecules that result from the replication of those described in (i) above.

Synthetic DNA segments which are likely to yield a potentially harmful polynucleotide or polypeptide (e.g., a toxin or a pharmacologically active agent) are considered as equivalent to their natural DNA counterpart. If the synthetic DNA segment is not expressed *in vivo* as a biologically active polynucleotide or polypeptide product, it is exempt from the *NIH Guidelines.*

Genomic DNA of plants and bacteria that have acquired a transposable element, even if the latter was donated from a recombinant vector no longer present, are not subject to the *NIH Guidelines* unless the transposon itself contains recombinant DNA.

Section I-C. General Applicability

Section I-C-1-a. All recombinant DNA research within the United States (U.S.) or its territories that is within the category of research described in either Section I-C-1-a-(1) or Section I-C-1-a-(2).

Section I-C-1-a-(1). Research that is conducted at or sponsored by an institution that receives any support for recombinant DNA research from NIH, including research performed directly by NIH. An individual who receives support for research involving recombinant DNA must be associated with or sponsored by an institution that assumes the responsibilities assigned in the *NIH Guidelines.*

Section I-C-1-a-(2). Research that involves testing in humans of materials containing recombinant DNA developed with NIH funds, if the institution that developed those materials sponsors or participates in those projects. Participation includes research collaboration or contractual agreements, not mere provision of research materials.

Section I-C-1-b. All recombinant DNA research performed abroad that is within the category of research described in either Section I-C-1-b-(1) or Section I-C-1-b-(2).

Section I-C-1-b-(1). Research supported by NIH funds.

Section I-C-1-b-(2). Research that involves testing in humans of materials containing recombinant DNA developed with NIH funds, if the institution that developed those materials sponsors or participates in those projects. Participation includes research collaboration or contractual agreements, not mere provision of research materials.

Section I-C-1-b-(3). If the host country has established rules for the conduct of recombinant DNA research, then the research must be in compliance with those rules. If the host country does not have such rules, the proposed research must be reviewed and approved by an NIH-approved Institutional Biosafety Committee or equivalent review body and accepted in writing by an appropriate national governmental authority of the host country. The safety practices that are employed abroad must be reasonably consistent with the *NIH Guidelines.*

Section I-D. Compliance with the *NIH Guidelines*

As a condition for NIH funding of recombinant DNA research, institutions shall ensure that such research conducted at or sponsored by the institution, irrespective of the source of funding, shall comply with the *NIH Guidelines.*

Information concerning noncompliance with the *NIH Guidelines* may be brought forward by any person. It should be delivered to both NIH/OBA and the relevant institution. The institution, generally through the Institutional Biosafety Committee, shall take appropriate action. The institution shall forward a complete report of the incident recommending any further action to the Office of Biotechnology Activities, National Institutes of Health, 6705 Rockledge Drive, Suite 750, MSC 7985, Bethesda, MD 20892-7985, 301-496-9838/301-496-9839 (fax) (for non-USPS mail, use Zip code 20817).

In cases where NIH proposes to suspend, limit, or terminate financial assistance because of noncompliance with the *NIH Guidelines,* applicable DHHS and Public Health Service procedures shall govern.

The policies on compliance are as follows:

Section I-D-1. All NIH-funded projects involving recombinant DNA techniques must comply with the *NIH Guidelines.* Non-compliance may result in: (i) suspension, limitation, or termination of financial assistance for the noncompliant NIH-funded research project and of NIH funds for other recombinant DNA research at the institution, or (ii) a requirement for prior NIH approval of any or all recombinant DNA projects at the institution.

Section I-D-2. All non-NIH funded projects involving recombinant DNA techniques conducted at or sponsored by an institution that receives NIH funds for projects involving such techniques must comply with the *NIH Guidelines.* Non-compliance may result in: (i) suspension, limitation, or termination of NIH funds for recombinant DNA research at the institution, or (ii) a requirement for prior NIH approval of any or all recombinant DNA projects at the institution.

Section I-E. General Definitions

The following terms, which are used throughout the *NIH Guidelines,* are defined as follows:

Section I-E-1. An "institution" is any public or private entity (including Federal, state, and local government agencies).

Section I-E-2. An "Institutional Biosafety Committee" is a committee that: (i) meets the requirements for membership specified in *Section IV-B-2, Institutional Biosafety Committee (IBC),* and (ii) reviews, approves, and oversees projects in accordance with the responsibilities defined in *Section IV-B-2, Institutional Biosafety Committee (IBC).*

Section I-E-3. The "Office of Biotechnology Activities (OBA)" is the office within the NIH that is responsible for: (i) reviewing and coordinating all activities relating to the *NIH Guidelines,* and (ii) performing other duties as defined in *Section IV-C-3, Office of Biotechnology Activities (OBA).*

Section I-E-4. The "Recombinant DNA Advisory Committee" is the public advisory committee that advises the Department of Health and Human Services (DHHS) Secretary, the DHHS Assistant Secretary for Health, and the NIH Director concerning recombinant DNA research. The RAC shall be constituted as specified in *Section IV-C-2, Recombinant DNA Advisory Committee (RAC).*

Section I-E-5. The "NIH Director" is the Director of the National Institutes of Health, or any other officer or employee of NIH to whom authority has been delegated.

Section I-E-6. "Deliberate release" is defined as a planned introduction of recombinant DNA-containing microorganisms, plants, or animals into the environment.

Section I-E-7. "Enrollment" is the process of obtaining informed consent from a potential research participant, or a designated legal guardian of the participant, to undergo a test or procedure associated with the gene transfer experiment.

Section I-E-8. A "serious adverse event" is any event occurring at any dose that results in any of the following outcomes: death, a life-threatening event, in-patient hospitalization or prolongation of existing hospitalization, a persistent or significant disability/incapacity, or a congenital anomaly/birth defect. Important medical events that may not result in death, be life-threatening, or require hospitalization also may be considered a serious adverse event when, upon the basis of appropriate medical judgment, they may jeopardize the human gene transfer research subject and may require medical or surgical intervention to prevent one of the outcomes listed in this definition.

Section I-E-9. An adverse event is "associated with the use of a gene transfer product" when there is a reasonable possibility that the event may have been caused by the use of that product.

Section I-E-10. An "unexpected serious adverse event" is any serious adverse event for which the specificity or severity is not consistent with the risk information available in the current investigator's brochure.

SECTION II.   SAFETY CONSIDERATIONS
Section II-A.   Risk Assessment

Section II-A-1.   Risk Groups

Risk assessment is ultimately a subjective process. The investigator must make an initial risk assessment based on the Risk Group (RG) of an agent (see *Appendix B, Classification of Human Etiologic Agents on the Basis of Hazard*). Agents are classified into four Risk Groups (RGs) according to their relative pathogenicity for healthy adult humans by the following criteria: (1) Risk Group 1 (RG1) agents are not associated with disease in healthy adult humans. (2) Risk Group 2 (RG2) agents are associated with human disease which is rarely serious and for which preventive or therapeutic interventions are *often* available. (3) Risk Group 3 (RG3) agents are associated with serious or lethal human disease for which preventive or therapeutic interventions *may be* available. (4) Risk Group 4 (RG4) agents are likely to cause serious or lethal human disease for which preventive or therapeutic interventions are *not usually* available.

Section II-A-2.   Criteria for Risk Groups
Classification of agents in *Appendix B, Classification of Human Etiologic Agents on the Basis of Hazard,* is based on the potential effect of a biological agent on a healthy human adult and does not account for instances in which an individual may have increased susceptibility to such agents, for example, preexisting diseases, medications, compromised immunity, pregnancy or breast feeding (which may increase exposure of infants to some agents).

Personnel may need periodic medical surveillance to ascertain fitness to perform certain activities; they may also need to be offered prophylactic vaccines and boosters (see *Section IV-B-1-f, Responsibilities of the Institution, General Information*).

Section II-A-3.   Comprehensive Risk Assessment
In deciding on the appropriate containment for an experiment, the initial risk assessment from *Appendix B, Classification of Human Etiologic Agents on the Basis of Hazard,* should be followed by a thorough consideration of the agent itself and how it is to be manipulated. Factors to be considered in determining the level of containment include agent factors such as: virulence, pathogenicity, infectious dose, environmental stability, route of spread, communicability, operations, quantity, availability of vaccine or treatment, and gene product effects such as toxicity, physiological activity, and allergenicity. Any strain that is known to be more hazardous than the parent (wild-type) strain should be considered for handling at a higher containment level. Certain attenuated strains or strains that have been demonstrated to have irreversibly lost known virulence factors may qualify for a reduction of the containment level compared to the Risk Group assigned to the parent strain (see *Section V-B, Footnotes and References of Sections I-IV*).

A final assessment of risk based on these considerations is then used to set the appropriate containment conditions for the experiment (see *Section II-B, Containment*). The containment level required may be equivalent to the Risk Group classification of the agent or it may be raised or lowered as a result of the above considerations. The Institutional Biosafety Committee must approve the risk assessment and the biosafety containment level for recombinant DNA experiments described in *Sections III-A, Experiments that Require Institutional Biosafety Committee Approval, RAC Review, and NIH Director Approval Before Initiation; III-B, Experiments that Require NIH/OBA and Institutional Biosafety Committee Approval Before Initiation; III-C, Experiments that Require Institutional Biosafety Committee and Institutional Review Board Approvals and NIH/OBA Registration Before Initiation; and III-D, Experiments that Require Institutional Biosafety Committee Approval Before Initiation.*

Careful consideration should be given to the types of manipulation planned for some higher Risk Group agents. For example, the RG2 dengue viruses may be cultured under the Biosafety Level (BL) 2 containment (see *Section II-B*); however, when such agents are used for animal inoculation or transmission studies, a higher containment level is recommended. Similarly, RG3 agents such as Venezuelan equine encephalomyelitis and yellow fever viruses should be handled at a higher containment level for animal inoculation and transmission experiments.

Individuals working with human immunodeficiency virus (HIV), hepatitis B virus (HBV) or other blood-borne pathogens should consult the applicable *Occupational Safety and Health Administration (OSHA)* regulation, 29 CFR 1910.1030, and OSHA publication 3127 (1996 revised). BL2 containment is recommended for activities involving all blood-contaminated clinical specimens, body fluids, and tissues from all humans, or from HIV- or HBV-infected or inoculated laboratory animals. Activities such as the production of research-laboratory scale quantities of HIV or other bloodborne pathogens, manipulating concentrated virus preparations, or conducting procedures that may produce droplets or aerosols, are performed in a BL2 facility using the additional practices and containment equipment recommended for BL3. Activities involving industrial scale volumes or preparations of concentrated HIV are conducted in a BL3 facility, or BL3 Large Scale if appropriate, using BL3 practices and containment equipment.

Exotic plant pathogens and animal pathogens of domestic livestock and poultry are restricted and may require special laboratory design, operation and containment features not addressed in *Biosafety in Microbiological and Biomedical Laboratories* (see *Section V-C, Footnotes and References of Sections I through IV*). For information regarding the importation, possession, or use of these agents see *Sections V-G and V-H, Footnotes and References of Sections I through IV.*

Section II-B.   Containment
Effective biological safety programs have been operative in a variety of laboratories for many years. Considerable information already exists about the design of

physical containment facilities and selection of laboratory procedures applicable to organisms carrying recombinant DNA (see *Section V-B, Footnotes and References of Sections I-IV*). The existing programs rely upon mechanisms that can be divided into two categories: (i) a set of standard practices that are generally used in microbiological laboratories; and (ii) special procedures, equipment, and laboratory installations that provide physical barriers that are applied in varying degrees according to the estimated biohazard. Four biosafety levels are described in *Appendix G, Physical Containment*. These biosafety levels consist of combinations of laboratory practices and techniques, safety equipment, and laboratory facilities appropriate for the operations performed and are based on the potential hazards imposed by the agents used and for the laboratory function and activity. Biosafety Level 4 provides the most stringent containment conditions, Biosafety Level 1 the least stringent.

Experiments involving recombinant DNA lend themselves to a third containment mechanism, namely, the application of highly specific biological barriers. Natural barriers exist that limit either: (i) the infectivity of a vector or vehicle (plasmid or virus) for specific hosts, or (ii) its dissemination and survival in the environment. Vectors, which provide the means for recombinant DNA and/or host cell replication, can be genetically designed to decrease, by many orders of magnitude, the probability of dissemination of recombinant DNA outside the laboratory (see *Appendix I, Biological Containment*).

Since these three means of containment are complementary, different levels of containment can be established that apply various combinations of the physical and biological barriers along with a constant use of standard practices. Categories of containment are considered separately in order that such combinations can be conveniently expressed in the *NIH Guidelines*.

Physical containment conditions within laboratories, described in *Appendix G, Physical Containment*, may not always be appropriate for all organisms because of their physical size, the number of organisms needed for an experiment, or the particular growth requirements of the organism. Likewise, biological containment for microorganisms described in *Appendix I, Biological Containment*, may not be appropriate for all organisms, particularly higher eukaryotic organisms. However, significant information exists about the design of research facilities and experimental procedures that are applicable to organisms containing recombinant DNA that is either integrated into the genome or into microorganisms associated with the higher organism as a symbiont, pathogen, or other relationship. This information describes facilities for physical containment of organisms used in non-traditional laboratory settings and special practices for limiting or excluding the unwanted establishment, transfer of genetic information, and dissemination of organisms beyond the intended location, based on both physical and biological containment principles. Research conducted in accordance with these conditions effectively confines the organism.

For research involving plants, four biosafety levels (BL1-P through BL4-P) are described in *Appendix P, Physical and Biological Containment for Recombinant DNA Research Involving Plants.* BL1-P is designed to provide a moderate level of containment for experiments for which there is convincing biological evidence that precludes the possibility of survival, transfer, or dissemination of recombinant DNA into the environment, or in which there is no recognizable and predictable risk to the environment in the event of accidental release. BL2-P is designed to provide a greater level of containment for experiments involving plants and certain associated organisms in which there is a recognized possibility of survival, transmission, or dissemination of recombinant DNA containing organisms, but the consequence of such an inadvertent release has a predictably minimal biological impact. BL3-P and BL4-P describe additional containment conditions for research with plants and certain pathogens and other organisms that require special containment because of their recognized potential for significant detrimental impact on managed or natural ecosystems. BL1-P relies upon accepted scientific practices for conducting research in most ordinary greenhouse or growth chamber facilities and incorporates accepted procedures for good pest control and cultural practices. BL1-P facilities and procedures provide a modified and protected environment for the propagation of plants and microorganisms associated with the plants and a degree of containment that adequately controls the potential for release of biologically viable plants, plant parts, and microorganisms associated with them. BL2-P and BL3-P rely upon accepted scientific practices for conducting research in greenhouses with organisms infecting or infesting plants in a manner that minimizes or prevents inadvertent contamination of plants within or surrounding the greenhouse. BL4-P describes facilities and practices known to provide containment of certain exotic plant pathogens.

For research involving animals, which are of a size or have growth requirements that preclude the use of conventional primary containment systems used for small laboratory animals, four biosafety levels (BL1-N through BL4-N) are described in *Appendix Q, Physical and Biological Containment for Recombinant DNA Research Involving Animals.* BL1-N describes containment for animals that have been modified by stable introduction of recombinant DNA, or DNA derived therefrom, into the germ-line (transgenic animals) and experiments involving viable recombinant DNA-modified microorganisms and is designed to eliminate the possibility of sexual transmission of the modified genome or transmission of recombinant DNA-derived viruses known to be transmitted from animal parent to offspring only by sexual reproduction. Procedures, practices, and facilities follow classical methods of avoiding genetic exchange between animals. BL2-N describes containment which is used for transgenic animals associated with recombinant DNA-derived organisms and is designed to eliminate the possibility of vertical or horizontal transmission. Procedures, practices, and facilities follow classical methods of avoiding genetic exchange between animals or controlling arthropod transmission. BL3-N and BL4-N describe higher levels of containment for research with certain transgenic animals involving agents which pose recognized hazard.

In constructing the *NIH Guidelines,* it was necessary to define boundary conditions for the different levels of physical and biological containment and for the classes of experiments to which they apply. These definitions do not take into account all existing and anticipated information on special procedures that will allow particular experiments to be conducted under different conditions than indicated here without affecting risk. Individual investigators and Institutional Biosafety Committees are urged to devise simple and more effective containment procedures and to submit recommended changes in the *NIH Guidelines* to permit the use of these procedures.

SECTION III. EXPERIMENTS COVERED BY THE *NIH GUIDELINES*

This section describes six categories of experiments involving recombinant DNA: (i) those that require Institutional Biosafety Committee (IBC) approval, RAC review, and NIH Director approval before initiation (see *Section III-A*), (ii) those that require NIH/OBA and Institutional Biosafety Committee approval before initiation (see *Section III-B*), (iii) those that require Institutional Biosafety Committee and Institutional Review Board approvals and RAC review before research participant enrollment (see *Section III-C*), (iv) those that require Institutional Biosafety Committee approval before initiation (see *Section III-D*), (v) those that require Institutional Biosafety Committee notification simultaneous with initiation (see *Section III-E*), and (vi) those that are exempt from the *NIH Guidelines* (see *Section III-F*).

Note: *If an experiment falls into Sections III-A, III-B, or III-C and one of the other sections, the rules pertaining to Sections III-A, III-B, or III-C shall be followed.* If an experiment falls into Section III-F and into either Sections III-D or III-E as well, the experiment is considered exempt from the *NIH Guidelines.*

Any change in containment level, which is different from those specified in the *NIH Guidelines,* may not be initiated without the express approval of NIH/OBA (see *Section IV-C-1-b-(2)* and its subsections, *Minor Actions*).

Section III-A.   Experiments that Require Institutional Biosafety Committee Approval, RAC Review, and NIH Director Approval Before Initiation

Section III-A-1.   Major Actions under the *NIH Guidelines*

Experiments considered as *Major Actions under the NIH Guidelines* cannot be initiated without submission of relevant information on the proposed experiment to the Office of Biotechnology Activities, National Institutes of Health, 6705

Rockledge Drive, Suite 750, MSC 7985, Bethesda, MD 20892-7985 (20817 for non-USPS mail), 301-496-9838, 301-496-9839 (fax), the publication of the proposal in the *Federal Register* for 15 days of comment, review by RAC, and specific approval by NIH. The containment conditions or stipulation requirements for such experiments will be recommended by RAC and set by NIH at the time of approval. Such experiments require Institutional Biosafety Committee approval before initiation. Specific experiments already approved are included in *Appendix D, Major Actions Taken under the NIH Guidelines,* which may be obtained from the Office of Biotechnology Activities, National Institutes of Health, 6705 Rockledge Drive, Suite 750, MSC 7985, Bethesda, MD 20892-7985 (20817 for non-USPS mail), 301-496-9838, 301-496-9839 (fax).

Section III-A-1-a. The deliberate transfer of a drug resistance trait to microorganisms that are not known to acquire the trait naturally (see *Section V-B, Footnotes and References of Sections I-IV*), if such acquisition could compromise the use of the drug to control disease agents in humans, veterinary medicine, or agriculture, will be reviewed by RAC.

Section III-B. Experiments that Require NIH/OBA and Institutional Biosafety Committee Approval Before Initiation

Experiments in this category cannot be initiated without submission of relevant information on the proposed experiment to NIH/OBA. The containment conditions for such experiments will be determined by NIH/OBA in consultation with ad hoc experts. Such experiments require Institutional Biosafety Committee approval before initiation (see *Section IV-B-2-b-(1), Institutional Biosafety Committee*).

GELSINGER V. UNIVERSITY OF PENNSYLVANIA

Jesse Gelsinger was an 18-year-old human research subject in a 1999 phase I safety trial at the University of Pennsylvania's Wistar Institute of Anatomy and Biology. Clinical trials were being conducted to evaluate the safety of a gene therapy technique. Gelsinger was generally healthy, although he suffered from a mild form of the metabolic disorder ornithine transcarbamylase (OTC) deficiency. He died four days after being treated with the experimental gene therapy. Researchers deviated from their FDA-approved protocol. The plaintiffs settled with the university for an undisclosed amount.

Text of *Gelsinger v. University of Pennyslvania*

> THIS IS NOT AN ARBITRATION MATTER. ASSESSMENT OF DAMAGES HEARING IS REQUIRED. JURY TRIAL OF TWELVE (12) PERSONS DEMANDED.

SHERMAN, SILVERSTEIN, KOHL,
ROSE & PODOLSKY
ALAN MILSTEIN/HARRIS POGUST

I.D. NOS. 38387/52721   **ATTORNEYS FOR PLAINTIFFS**

Fairway Corporate Center
4300 Haddonfield Road - Suite 311
Pennsauken, NJ 08109
(856) 662-0700

SALTZ, MONGELUZZI, BARRETT & BENDESKY, P.C.
ROBERT J. MONGELUZZI/LARRY BENDESKY

I.D. NOS. 36283/51026   **ATTORNEYS FOR PLAINTIFFS**

34th Floor
1650 Market Street
Philadelphia, PA 19103
(215) 496-8282

JOHN GELSINGER as ADMINISTRATOR AND PERSONAL REPRESENTATIVE OF THE ESTATE OF JESSE GELSINGER AND PAUL GELSINGER, in his own right,	PHILADELPHIA COUNTY COURT OF COMMON PLEAS TRIAL DIVISION
Plaintiffs	TERM, 2000
THE TRUSTEES OF THE UNIVERSITY OF PENNSYLVANIA, JAMES WILSON, M.D., GENOVO, INC., STEVEN RAPER, M.D. MARK BATSHAW, M.D., WILLIAM KELLEY, M.D. CHILDREN'S HOPSITAL OF PHILADELPHIA, CHILDREN'S NATIONAL MEDICAL CENTER, AND ARTHUR CAPLAN, Ph.D.	No.
Defendants	

COMPLAINT—CIVIL ACTION

John Gelsinger, as Administrator and Personal Representative of the Estate of
Jesse Gelsinger, and Paul Gelsinger in his own right, claim of defendants, both

jointly and severally, a sum in excess of Fifty Thousand Dollars ($50,000.00) in compensatory and punitive damages, upon causes of action whereof the following are true statements:

1. On September 17, 1999, Jesse Gelsinger, an 18-year-old young man died while participating in a gene transfer experiment at the Institute for Human Gene Therapy ("IHGT") located at the University of Pennsylvania.

2. At the time of his death, Jesse suffered from a mild form of ornithine transcarbamylase deficiency ("OTC"), a rare metabolic disorder, which was controlled with a low-protein diet and drugs. Jesse volunteered to participate in the experiment, knowing it would not benefit his condition in the least, because he was led to believe his participation held little risk and would directly benefit yet to be born infants with OTC.

3. While at IHGT, Jesse Gelsinger was infused with trillions of particles of an adenovirus vector, which was developed at the University for the purpose of transferring OTC genes.

4. The adenovirus vector used by the defendants was known to be more toxic than other vectors used in gene transfer.

5. When Jesse Gelsinger received the vector, he suffered a chain reaction including jaundice, a blood-clotting disorder, kidney failure, lung failure and brain death.

6. On September 17, 1999, Jesse Gelsinger died as a direct result of the carelessness, negligence, recklessness and wanton and willful conduct of defendants as described in detail below.

7. Plaintiff, John Gelsinger, is an individual residing at 47 Tallowood Drive, Medford, New Jersey 08055.

8. Plaintiff, John Gelsinger, was duly appointed Personal Representative of the Estate of Jesse Gelsinger by Issuance of Letters dated March 22, 2000 by the Superior Court of Arizona, Pima County.

9. Plaintiff, Paul Gelsinger is a citizen and resident of the State of Arizona, residing at 6901 East Hawthorne Street, Tucson, Arizona 85710. Paul Gelsinger is the father of Jesse Gelsinger.

10. Defendant, the Trustees of the University of Pennsylvania ("the University") is an educational institution, incorporated in the Commonwealth of Pennsylvania, with its principal place of business located at 3450 Hamilton Walk, Philadelphia, PA 19104. IHGT is an institute within and under the control of the University, which conducts substantial, systematic, continuous and regular business in the County of Philadelphia, Commonwealth of Pennsylvania.

11. Defendant, James Wilson, M.D., is a citizen and resident of the Commonwealth of Pennsylvania residing at 1350 N. Avignon Drive, Gladwyne, PA 19104.

12. Defendant, Genovo, Inc., is a corporation organized and existing by and under the laws of the State of Delaware with its principal office and place

of business located at 512 Elmwood Avenue, Elmwood Court Two, Sharon Hill, PA 19079. Genovo currently provides nearly a quarter of the budget for the IHGT, and conducts substantial, systematic, continuous and regular business in the County of Philadelphia, Commonwealth of Pennsylvania.

13. At all times relevant hereto, Dr. Wilson was the founder of defendant Genovo, a biotech company. At all times relevant hereto, Dr. Wilson controlled up to thirty percent (30%) of the Genovo stock.

14. Genovo agreed to provide the IHGT with over four million dollars a year for five years to conduct genetic research and experimentation.

15. In lieu of up-front payments to the University, Genovo transferred five percent (5%) equity ownership to the University.

16. In return for Genovo's sponsorship of genetic research and experimentation, the University agreed to grant Genovo licenses for the lung and liver applications for existing technologies developed by defendant, Dr. Wilson.

17. Defendant, Genovo, retained an option to negotiate for licenses for any future developments by defendants, IHGT and/or Dr. Wilson.

18. The proposed licenses between the defendants included full patent reimbursement, milestone payments and royalties on product sales.

19. The shareholders of Genovo include numerous past and present University and/or IHGT employees.

20. Dr. Wilson is a duly licensed practicing physician in the Commonwealth of Pennsylvania and, at all times mentioned herein and material hereto, was the director of the IHGT and an attending physician on the staff of the University of Pennsylvania Hospital. At all times mentioned herein and material hereto, Dr. Wilson was an agent, servant, representative and employee of the University.

21. At the time of the occurrence of the incidents described herein, Dr. Wilson was also acting as an agent, servant, workman, and employee of Genovo.

22. Defendant Steven Raper, M.D., is a duly licensed physician in the Commonwealth of Pennsylvania, residing at 127 Kynlyn Road, Radnor, PA 19087 and with offices located at 3450 Hamilton Walk, Philadelphia, Pennsylvania and, at all times mentioned herein and material hereto, was an attending physician on the staff of the University of Pennsylvania Hospital and the IHGT. At all times mentioned herein and material hereto, Dr. Raper was an agent, servant, representative and employee of both the University and the IHGT.

23. Defendant Mark L. Batshaw, M.D., is a duly licensed practicing physician in Washington, D.C., with offices located at Childrens National Medical Center, 111 Michigan Avenue, Washington, D.C. 20010, and, at all times mentioned herein and material hereto, was an attending physician on the staff of the University of Pennsylvania Hospital and the IHGT. At all times mentioned herein and material hereto, Dr. Batshaw was an agent, servant,

representative and employee of the University, Children's Hospital of Philadelphia, Children's National Medical Center and the IHGT.

24. Defendant, Children's Hospital of Philadelphia (CHOP), is a corporation and medical center, existing by and under the laws of the Commonwealth of Pennsylvania with its principal place of business at 34th Street and Civic Center Boulevard, Philadelphia, PA 19104-4399.

25. At all times mentioned herein and material hereto, defendant, CHOP, held itself and its agents, servants, workers, representatives, physicians, nurses, staff, contractors, medical personnel and employees out to be skillful and qualified to administer medical care and treatment.

26. Defendant, Children's National Medical Center, is a corporation and medical center, existing by and under the law of the District of Columbia with its principal place of business located at 111 Michigan Avenue, Washington, D.C. 20010.

27. At all times mentioned herein and material hereto, defendant, Children's National Medical Center, held itself and its agents, servants, workers, representatives, physicians, nurses, staff, contractors, medical personnel and employees out to be skillful and qualified to administer medical care and treatment.

28. Defendant, William N. Kelley, M.D. ("Dr. Kelley"), is the former dean of the University of Pennsylvania Medical School and chief executive of its health system.

29. Dr. Kelley arrived at the University in 1989.

30. At the time of his arrival at the University, Dr. Kelley and two colleagues had already applied for a patent which Dr. Kelley claimed "is a broad gene therapy patent which involves any DNA or piece thereof."

31. This patent enabled Dr. Kelley to collect royalties, should gene therapy research using the replication-defective adeno-viral ("RDAd") vectors prove to be effective.

32. In 1992, Dr. Wilson founded Genovo, Inc., a company in the business of gene transfer research and development.

33. In the spring of 1993, Dr. Wilson was recruited by Dr. Kelley to come to the University and be the director of the IHGT.

34. Defendant, Dr. Kelley, approved Dr. Wilson's OTC gene transfer experiments involving a RDAd vector, a vector similar to the one patented by defendants, Dr. Kelley, Genovo and Dr. Wilson.

35. Defendants, Dr. Kelley, Genovo, and Dr. Wilson all stood to gain financially from the successful use of RDAd vectors.

36. Defendants, the University and/or IHGT, stood to gain financially through their equity stake in Genovo from the successful use of RDAd vectors.

37. Defendant, Arthur Caplan, Ph.D., is the director of the Bioethics Department of the University of Pennsylvania, with offices located at the University of Pennsylvania, 3401 Market Street, Suite 320, Philadelphia, PA 19104-3319.

38. Defendant, Arthur Caplan, was appointed as Trustee Professor of Bioethics in the Department of Molecular and Cellular Engineering, which defendant, Dr. Wilson, chaired.

39. Defendant, Arthur Caplan, was consulted to determine the ethical complications surrounding the OTC gene transfer experiment.

40. The IHGT agreed to provide funding, in the amount of approximately $25,000.00 per year, for a bioethics faculty position.

41. The gene therapy study was initially designed to enroll terminally ill infants as subjects for the experiment.

42. Defendant, Arthur Caplan, advised defendants, Drs. Wilson, Batshaw and Raper, that parents of terminally ill children were incapable of giving an informed consent and suggested that the gene transfer experiment be performed on otherwise healthy, adults with a mild, medically manageable, form of OTC.

43. Defendant, Arthur Caplan, was quoted subsequent to the death of Jesse Gelsinger as saying, "Not only is it sad that Jesse Gelsinger died, there was never a chance that anybody would benefit from these experiments. They are safety studies. They are not therapeutic in goal. *If I gave it to you, we would try to see if you died, too,* or if you did OK."

44. Defendant, Arthur Caplan, was also quoted in relation to gene therapy as follows, "*If you cured anybody, you'd publish it in a religious journal. It would be a miracle.* The researchers wouldn't say that. But I'm telling you. If you cured anybody from a phase one gene therapy trial, it would be a miracle. *All you're doing is you're saying, I've got this vector, I want to see if it can deliver the gene where I want it to go without killing, or hurting or having side effects.*"

45. The Internal Review Board (IRB) of defendant, CHOP, reviewed and approved the protocol for the OTC gene transfer experiment.

46. Hematologists for defendant, CHOP, were consulted regarding the gene transfer experiment.

47. In September of 1994, the stock of Genovo was distributed to the founders of Genovo.

48. These founders include Ms. Marian Grossman who became the Director of the Human Applications Laboratory of the IHGT; Mr. Dennis Berman; Dr. Barbara Handelin who was Genovo's Chief Scientific Officer and the wife of a University faculty member in Dr. Wilson's department; and Dr. Wilson.

49. Upon his arrival at the University, Dr. Wilson had numerous patents which, like the patent held by Dr. Kelley, involved the use of the RDAD vector for gene transfer.

50. In late 1994, the University began discussions with Dr. Wilson concerning his being employed by the University. At the same time the University began discussions with Dr. Wilson concerning an arrangement between the University and Genovo.

51. During this time, the University's Conflicts of Interest Standing Committee ("CISC") held meetings during which the issue of what, if any, conflicts of interest would arise if an agreement was entered into between the University, Genovo and Dr. Wilson.

52. During the meeting of the CISC held on February 6, 1995, committee members asserted that a conflict of interest may exist regarding the relationship between the University, Dr. Wilson, and Genovo.

53. The CISC, an agent of the University, was expressly aware that a conflict of interest would exist if Dr. Wilson were permitted to conduct experiments at IHGT which, if successful, would directly benefit Dr. Wilson and Genovo financially.

54. Despite such express knowledge of the dangers such a conflict of interest would present, the University accepted the Genovo arrangement and allowed Dr. Wilson to conduct experiments at IHGT.

55. Jesse Gelsinger was first diagnosed with OTC at the age of two.

56. OTC is a rare metabolic disorder which affects the body's ability to break down ammonia, a normal byproduct of metabolism.

57. Over the next sixteen years, Jesse Gelsinger controlled the disease with a low-protein diet and medication.

58. In September 1998, Jesse was told by his treating physician of an OTC gene transfer trial which was being conducted at the IHGT.

59. On June 22, 1999, Jesse and Paul Gelsinger went to the IHGT where they met Dr. Raper who performed blood and liver-function tests to determine whether Jesse was eligible for the gene transfer trial. Jesse was to receive no financial compensation for participating in the trial.

60. Between June 22, 1999 and September 9, 1999, Jesse and Paul Gelsinger reviewed documents and had discussions with Drs. Raper and Batshaw which purportedly were to provide certain information necessary to make an informed decision as to whether Jesse was going to take part in and was an appropriate candidate for the gene transfer trial.

61. Such documents and discussions were materially misleading and deceptive because, among other things:

   a. the risks of the toxic effects of the injection of the adenovirus particles were understated;

   b. no mention was made that monkeys injected with the virus had become ill and/or died;

   c. no mention was made that patients who had previously participated in the trial suffered serious adverse effects;

   d. the representation was made that IHGT had achieved certain efficacy with respect to the treatment of OTC; and

   e. the extent to which Dr. Wilson and the University had a conflict of interest was not adequately disclosed.

62. The effects of such misrepresentations and nondisclosure were that Jesse and Paul Gelsinger believed the risks of injection of the adenovirus vector

were minimal and the potential benefits of Jesse's participation to the future treatment of OTC patients in the study were enormous.

63. On September 9, 1999, Jesse returned to Philadelphia to begin the gene transfer trial.

64. Jesse was scheduled to be the last of three patients in the sixth cohort in the trial.

65. On September 13, 1999, Jesse was taken to the interventional-radiology suite where he was sedated and strapped to a table while a team of radiologists threaded two catheters into his groin.

66. At approximately 10:30 a.m., Dr. Raper drew 30 milliliters of the vector and injected it into Jesse.

67. The procedure was completed at approximately 12:30 p.m.

68. On the evening of September 13, 1999, Jesse was sick to his stomach and had a fever of 104.5 degrees.

69. The following morning Jesse seemed disoriented.

70. When Dr. Raper examined Jesse the morning of September 14, 1999, he noticed that Jesse's eyes were yellow.

71. Blood tests performed on September 14, 1999, indicated that Jesse's bilirubin was four times the normal level.

72. The symptoms that Jesse was experiencing were similar to those defendants had seen in the monkeys that had been given a similar vector.

73. By the afternoon of September 14, 1999, Jesse had slipped into a coma.

74. At 11:30 p.m. on September 14, 1999, Jesse's ammonia level was 393 micromoles per deciliter of blood. The normal level is 35 micromoles.

75. Thereafter, the doctors placed Jesse on dialysis.

76. Initially, Jesse's condition improved but soon began to deteriorate.

77. After consultation between Drs. Wilson, Raper and Batshaw, the doctors decided to perform extracorporeal membrane oxygenation.

78. On September 16, 1999, Jesse's kidneys stopped making urine and he began to suffer from multiple organ system failure.

79. On the evening of September 16, 1999, Jesse was bloated beyond recognition; his ears and eyes had swollen shut.

80. On the morning of September 17, 1999, tests indicated that Jesse was brain-dead.

81. On September 17, 1999, the ECMO machine was shut off and Jesse was pronounced dead at 2:30 p.m.

82. The cause of Jesse's death was attributed to acute respiratory distress and multiple-organ failure, both of which were the direct result of injection of the adenovirus vector.

83. After Jesse's death, the FDA determined there were numerous violations of FDA guidelines by the defendants. Some of these violations were:

   a. failing to tell the National Institute of Health Recombinant DNA Advisory Committee ("the RAC") of a change in the way the virus was to be delivered to patients;

b. changing the informed consent form from what had been approved by the FDA by removing information concerning the death or illness of several monkeys during a similar study;

c. failing to report to the FDA that patients prior to Jesse suffered significant liver toxicity which required that the study be put on hold;

d. failing to follow the study protocol which mandated that in each cohort at least two women be subject to injection before any male;

e. admitting Jesse in the trial when his blood ammonia level on the day before he received the gene transfer exceeded the limit set out in the FDA protocol; and

f. allowing the vectors to sit and/or be stored on lab shelves for 25 months before being tested in animals, making them less potent than they could have been. The vectors administered to the plaintiff's decedent were only stored for two months. The 25-month storage in turn, may have resulted in an underestimation of the vectors potency in humans. Additionally, the animals who received the vector stored for 25-months would have been given a dose of vector from 52.2% to 65.3% below the vector dose specified in the FDA protocol.

COUNT I—WRONGFUL DEATH

JOHN GELSINGER, AS ADMINISTRATOR AND PERSONAL REPRESENTATIVE OF THE ESTATE OF JESSE GELSINGER v. THE TRUSTEES OF THE UNIVERSITY OF PENNSYLVANIA, CHILDREN'S HOSPITAL OF PHILADELPHIA, CHILDREN'S NATIONAL MEDICAL CENTER, JAMES WILSON, M.D., GENOVO, INC., STEVEN RAPER, M.D. MARK BATSHAW, M.D., WILLIAM N. *KELLEY, M.D., AND ARTHUR CAPLAN, Ph.D.*

84. Plaintiffs incorporate by reference paragraphs 1 through 83 as if fully set forth at length herein.

85. At all times mentioned herein and material hereto, the defendants, and each of them respectively, jointly and severally, were charged with the professional responsibility of rendering proper care and treatment to Jesse Gelsinger, of properly and carefully examining him in order to determine his condition and eligibility for the gene transfer trial, of properly and carefully administering the gene transfer protocol in a careful and prudent fashion, and of assuring that proper medical care and attention were provided during all periods of time during which he remained under said defendants' care and treatment.

86. As a result of the careless, negligent and reckless conduct of the defendants herein, Jesse Gelsinger was caused to suffer excruciating and agonizing pain and discomfort and ultimately died as a result of defendants' conduct.

87. Defendants together, and each of them respectively, jointly and severally, by and through their separate and respective agents, servants, workmen, representatives, physicians, nurses, staff, contractors, medical personnel, medical assistants and employees were careless, negligent and reckless in:
   a. failing to properly and adequately evaluate Jesse Gelsinger's condition and eligibility for the gene transfer trial;
   b. failing to properly diagnose Jessie Gelsinger's condition subsequent to the administration of the gene transfer;
   c. failing to perform proper and adequate testing for his condition;
   d. failing to properly and adequately treat his condition;
   e. failing to properly and adequately care for his condition;
   f. failing to monitor his ammonia levels both during and after the administration of the gene transfer;
   g. failing to provide and afford proper and careful medical care and treatment;
   h. failing to perform proper and careful medical practices and procedures in accordance with the standards prevailing in the community in which defendants practiced at the time;
   i. failing to properly care for his condition under all of the circumstances;
   j. caring for Jesse Gelsinger in a negligent and improper manner;
   k. failing to properly monitor his condition both prior to and subsequent to the performance of the gene transfer procedure;
   l. failing to use a proper, adequate and safe vector for gene transfer;
   m. failing to inform Jesse Gelsinger of all the risks of performing the gene transfer procedure so as to afford him with the opportunity to make an informed decision as to the performance of said procedure;
   n. failing to properly and timely observe, discover, diagnose, treat and care for his condition;
   o. failing to conform to the standard of care and treatment prevailing in the medical community in which defendants practiced at the time in conducting gene transfer;
   p. failing to exercise reasonable care under all of the circumstances, in accordance with the accepted practices and procedures in the medical community in which defendants practiced;
   q. failing to follow and abide by guidelines set forth by various governmental agencies; and
   r. acting negligently per se.
88. As a direct and proximate result of the carelessness, negligence, gross negligence, recklessness and willful and wanton conduct of defendants, and each of them respectively, jointly and severally, by and through their separate and respective agents, servants, workmen, representatives, physicians, nurses, staff, contractors, medical personnel and employees, Jesse Gelsinger was caused to sustain serious and excruciating personal injuries which ultimately led to his death. Jesse Gelsinger died as a result of acute respiratory distress and multiple-organ failure. He was caused to suffer agonizing

aches, pains and mental anguish; he sustained loss of enjoyment of life and loss of life's pleasures. As a result of his wrongful death he has been prevented from performing all of his usual duties, occupations, recreational activities and avocation all to his and his beneficiaries' loss and detriment.

89. By conducting themselves as aforesaid, defendants increased the risk of harm, thereby causing the wrongful death of Jesse Gelsinger.

90. As a direct and proximate result of the foregoing, decedent's wrongful death beneficiaries suffered, are suffering from an indefinite period of time in the future damages, injuries and losses, including, but not limited to, a loss of financial support, and the beneficiaries have been wrongfully deprived of the contributions they would have received from Jesse Gelsinger, including monies which decedent would have provided for such items such as clothing, shelter, food, medical care and education.

91. As a direct and proximate result of the foregoing, decedent's wrongful death beneficiaries would have been, continue to be and will be in the future wrongfully deprived of large and various sums of money which decedent would have contributed to their support.

92. As a direct and proximate result of the foregoing, decedent's wrongful death beneficiaries incurred or have been caused to incur and paid large and various expenses including funeral, burial and estate administration.

93. Plaintiff makes claim, on behalf of decedent's heirs-at-law and next of kin, for the loss of love, affection, services, earnings, support and all other damages recoverable under the Wrongful Death Statute of the Commonwealth of Pennsylvania.

WHEREFORE, John Gelsinger, as Administrator and Personal Representative of the Estate of Jesse Gelsinger, claim of defendants, and each of them respectively, jointly and severally, compensatory damages in excess of Fifty-thousand Dollars ($50,000.00), delay damages pursuant to Pa. R.C.P. 238, interest and allowable costs of suit.

COUNT II—SURVIVAL ACTION

JOHN GELSINGER, AS ADMINISTRATOR AND PERSONAL REPRESENTATIVE OF THE ESTATE OF JESSE GELSINGER v. THE TRUSTEES OF THE UNIVERSITY OF PENNSYLVANIA, CHILDREN'S HOSPITAL OF PHILADELPHIA, CHILDREN'S NATIONAL MEDICAL CENTER, JAMES WILSON, M.D., GENOVO, INC., STEVEN RAPER, M.D. MARK BATSHAW, M.D., WILLIAM N. KELLEY, M.D., AND ARTHUR CAPLAN, Ph.D.

94. Plaintiffs incorporate by reference paragraphs 1 through 93 as if fully set forth at length herein.

95. As a direct and proximate result of the foregoing, Jesse Gelsinger, has been, is being and will be in the future wrongfully deprived of earnings and the right to earn a living.

96. To address the foregoing, the Estate of Jesse Gelsinger, is entitled to recover in this action an amount equal to the gross amount decedent would have earned between the date of his death and the end of his life expectancy, subject to his cost of maintenance.

WHEREFORE, John Gelsinger, as Administrator and Personal Representative of the Estate of Jesse Gelsinger, claim of defendants, and each of them respectively, compensatory damages in excess of Fifty-thousand Dollars ($50,000.00), delay damages pursuant to Pa. R.C.P. 238, interest and allowable costs of suit.

COUNT III—STRICT PRODUCTS LIABILITY

**JOHN GELSINGER, AS ADMINISTRATOR
AND PERSONAL REPRESENTATIVE OF THE
ESTATE OF JESSE GELSINGER v. THE TRUSTEES
OF THE UNIVERSITY OF PENNSYLVANIA,
*JAMES WILSON, M.D., GENOVO, INC.***

97. Plaintiffs incorporate by reference paragraphs 1 through 96 as if fully set forth at length herein.

98. Defendants, Genovo, Inc. and James Wilson, M.D., designed, manufactured and supplied the adenovirus vector which ultimately caused the death of plaintiff's decedent, Jesse Gelsinger.

99. Defendant, IHGT, as a unit of the University, supplied the adenovirus vector which ultimately caused the death of plaintiff's decedent, Jesse Gelsinger.

100. The United States Patent issued to Defendant, Wilson, for the adenovirus vector describes the vector as "The present invention provides a unique recombinant adenovirus capable of delivering transgenes to target cells, as well as the components for production of the unique virus and methods for the use of the virus to treat a variety of genetic disorders. . . . This novel recombinant virus is produced by use of an adenovirus-based vector production system containing two components: (1) a shuttle vector that comprises adenovirus *cis*-elements necessary for replication and virion encapsidation and is deleted of all viral genes, which vector carries a reporter or therapeutic mini-gene and (2) a helper adenovirus which, alone or with a packaging of cell line, is capable of providing all of the viral gene products necessary for a productive viral infection when co-transfected with the shuttle vector . . . The methods of producing this viral vector from these components include both a novel means of packaging of an adenoviral/transgene containing vector into a virus, and a novel method for the subsequent separation of the helper virus from the newly formed recombinant virus."

101. IHGT, Dr. Wilson and Genovo breached their duties and obligations to plaintiffs by various sections of the *Restatement of Torts,* 2d, including Section 402(a) and are liable for causing injuries to Jesse Gelsinger for the following reasons:

   a. designing, manufacturing, selling and/or distributing a product in a defective condition;

   b. designing, manufacturing, selling and/or distributing a product which was unreasonably dangerous;

   c. designing, manufacturing, selling and/or distributing a product which was not safe for normal use and consumption;

   d. failing to have adequate warnings on the product;

   e. failing to warn users of the dangers inherent in using this product;

   f. designing, manufacturing, selling and/or distributing a product which could have been produced and manufactured more safely;

   g. designing, manufacturing, selling and/or distributing a product wherein it was foreseeable that someone would be harmed by the product's use;

   h. designing, manufacturing, selling and/or distributing a product which was not safe for its intended use;

   i. designing, manufacturing, selling and/or distributing a product which was lacking of one or more elements necessary to make it safe for its intended use;

   j. designing, manufacturing, selling and/or distributing a product which was defective and which could cause injury to the user;

   k. failing to ensure that ultimate users were advised of the dangers of said product;

   l. failing to exercise reasonable care in the design of this product;

   m. failing to exercise reasonable care in the distribution of this product;

   n. failing to adequately and properly test this product;

   o. failing to use reasonable care under the circumstances;

   p. delivering a product which was defective and could cause injury to the user;

   q. producing a product which was defective and could cause injury to the user;

   r. supplying a product which was defective and could cause injury to the user;

   s. knowing of prior adverse reaction to the adenovirus and failing to inform the user of these adverse reactions;

   t. failing to adequately and properly test the product after its design and manufacture;

   u. failing to investigate and analyze prior adverse reactions information in order to warn and/or notify ultimate users of the product defects and dangers;

   v. violating applicable sections of the *Restatement of Torts, 2d;*

   w. engaging in other acts regarding the manufacturing, designing, testing, preparing, producing, and distributing this product as will be learned in discovery.

102. By conducting themselves as aforesaid, defendants increased the risk of harm, thereby causing the injuries and wrongful death of Jesse Gelsinger.

103. As a direct and proximate result of the foregoing, decedent's wrongful death beneficiaries suffered, are suffering for an indefinite period of time in the future damages, injuries and losses, including but not limited to, a loss of financial support, and the beneficiaries have been wrongfully deprived of the contributions they would have received from decedent, Jesse Gelsinger, including monies which decedent would have provided for such items as clothing, shelter, food, medical care and education.

104. As a direct and proximate result of the foregoing, decedent's wrongful death beneficiaries would have been, continue to be and will be in the future wrongfully deprived of large and various sums of money which decedent would have contributed to their support.

105. As a direct and proximate result of the foregoing, decedent's wrongful death beneficiaries incurred or have been caused to incur and paid large and various expenses various funeral, burial and estate administration.

106. Plaintiff makes claim, on behalf of decedent's heirs-at-law and next-of-kin, for the loss of love, affection, companionship, services, earnings, support and all other damages recoverable under the Wrongful Death Statute of the Commonwealth of Pennsylvania.

107. Plaintiff makes claim, on behalf of his decedent's heirs-at-law and next-of-kin, for all damages recoverable under the Survival Statute of the Commonwealth of Pennsylvania.

WHEREFORE, John Gelsinger, as Administrator and Personal Representative of the Estate of Jesse Gelsinger, claim of defendants, and each of them respectively, jointly and severally, compensatory damages in excess of Fifty-thousand Dollars ($50,000.00), delay damages pursuant to Pa. R.C.P. 238, interest and allowable costs of suit.

COUNT IV—INTENTIONAL ASSAULT AND BATTERY, LACK OF INFORMED CONSENT

JOHN GELSINGER, AS ADMINISTRATOR AND PERSONAL REPRESENTATIVE OF THE ESTATE OF JESSE GELSINGER v. THE TRUSTEES OF THE UNIVERSITY OF PENNSYLVANIA, CHILDREN'S HOSPITAL OF PENNSYLVANIA, JAMES WILSON, M.D., STEVEN RAPER, M.D. AND MARK *BATSHAW, M.D.*

108. Plaintiffs incorporate by reference paragraphs 1 through 107 as if fully set forth at length herein.

109. Defendants, and each of them respectively, failed to inform plaintiff's decedent, Jesse Gelsinger, of the risks of all treatment, care, therapy and procedures performed upon him so as to afford plaintiff's decedent the opportunity to make an informed decision as to the performance of said procedures.
110. The lack of informed consent includes, but is not limited to:
    a. understating the risks of the toxic effects of the injection of the adenovirus particles;
    b. failing to inform plaintiff's decedent regarding the fact that monkeys injected with the virus had become ill and/or died;
    c. failing to inform plaintiff's decedent that patients who had previously participated in the trial suffered serious adverse effects;
    d. misrepresenting the fact that prior participants in the study had achieved certain efficacy with respect to the treatment of OTC;
    e. failing to adequately disclose the extent to which Dr. Wilson and the University had a conflict of interest;
    f. failing to adequately disclose the financial interest that Dr. Wilson and the University had in relation to the study; and
    g. allowing the vectors to sit and/or be stored on lab shelves for 25 months before being tested in animals, making them less potent then they could have been. The vectors administered to the plaintiff's decedent were only stored for two months. The 25 month storage in turn, may have resulted in an underestimation of the vectors potency in humans. Additionally, the animals who received the vector stored for 25 months would have been given a dose of vector from 52.2% to 65.3% below the vector dose specified in the FDA protocol.
111. As a result of the intentional tortious conduct of all the defendants named herein, and each of them respectively, by and through their separate and respective agents, servants, workmen, representatives, physicians, nurses, staff, contractors, medical personnel and employees, plaintiff's decedent, Jesse Gelsinger, was caused to suffer severe and agonizing personal injuries and pain and suffering which resulted in his untimely death on September 17, 1999.
112. As a result of the intentional tortious conduct of all defendants named herein, by and through their separate and respective agents, servants, workmen, representatives, physicians, nurses, staff, contractors, medical personnel and employees, said decedent's heirs-at-law and next of kin have in the past been and will in the future continue to be deprived of the earnings, comfort, society and companionship of their said decedent, all to their great loss and detriment.
113. As a direct and proximate result of the foregoing, decedent's wrongful death beneficiaries suffered, are suffering for an indefinite period of time in the future damages, injuries and losses, including but not limited to, a loss

of financial support, and the beneficiaries have been wrongfully deprived of the contributions they would have received from decedent, Jesse Gelsinger, including monies which decedent would have provided for such items as clothing, shelter, food, medical care and education.

114. As a direct and proximate result of the foregoing, decedent's wrongful death beneficiaries would have been, continue to be and will be in the future wrongfully deprived of large and various sums of money which decedent would have contributed to their support.

115. As a direct and proximate result of the foregoing, decedent's wrongful death beneficiaries incurred or have been caused to incur and paid large and various expenses various funeral, burial and estate administration.

116. Plaintiff makes claim, on behalf of decedent's heirs-at-law and next-of-kin, for the loss of love, affection, services, earnings, support and all other damages recoverable under the Wrongful Death Statute of the Commonwealth of Pennsylvania.

117. Plaintiff makes claim, on behalf of his decedent's heirs-at-law and next-of-kin, for all damages recoverable under the Survival Statute of the Commonwealth of Pennsylvania.

WHEREFORE, John Gelsinger, as Administrator and Personal Representative of the Estate of Jesse Gelsinger, claim of defendants, and each of them respectively, jointly and severally, compensatory damages in excess of Fifty-thousand Dollars ($50,000.00), delay damages pursuant to Pa. R.C.P. 238, interest and allowable costs of suit.

COUNT V—INTENTIONAL AND NEGLIGENT INFLICTION OF EMOTIONAL DISTRESS

JOHN GELSINGER, AS ADMINISTRATOR AND PERSONAL REPRESENTATIVE OF THE ESTATE OF JESSE GELSINGER v. THE TRUSTEES OF THE UNIVERSITY OF PENNSYLVANIA, CHILDREN'S HOSPITAL OF PHILADELPHIA, CHILDREN'S NATIONAL MEDICAL CENTER, JAMES WILSON, M.D., GENOVO, INC., STEVEN RAPER, M.D., MARK BATSHAW, M.D., WILLIAM N. *KELLEY, M.D., AND ARTHUR CAPLAN, Ph.D.*

118. Plaintiffs incorporate by reference paragraphs 1 through 117 inclusive, as if fully set forth at length herein.

119. Defendants engaged in the conduct described above and willfully, recklessly and/or negligently caused Paul Gelsinger severe emotional distress.

120. The conduct of defendants in making false statements to Paul Gelsinger, knowing he would rely on these statements in advising his son to participate

in the IHGT gene transfer trial which ultimately and directly resulted in his son's death, has caused emotional harm to Paul Gelsinger, and was extreme and outrageous.

121. Paul Gelsinger has suffered severe emotional distress as a result of the conduct of the defendants.

122. Defendants' actions were willful and/or reckless thus entitling plaintiffs to punitive damages.

WHEREFORE, Paul Gelsinger claims of defendants, and each of them respectively, jointly and severally, compensatory damages in excess of Fifty-thousand Dollars ($50,000.00), delay damages pursuant to Pa. R.C.P. 238, interest and allowable costs of suit.

COUNT VI—COMMON LAW FRAUD/INTENTIONAL MISREPRESENTATION

JOHN GELSINGER, AS ADMINISTRATOR AND PERSONAL REPRESENTATIVE OF THE ESTATE OF JESSE GELSINGER AND PAUL GELSINGER v. THE TRUSTEES OF THE UNIVERSITY OF PENNSYLVANIA, JAMES WILSON, M.D., *GENOVO, INC., STEVEN RAPER, M.D. AND MARK BATSHAW, M.D.*

123. Plaintiffs incorporate by reference paragraphs 1 through 122 as if fully set forth at length herein.

124. Defendants made the following intentional misrepresentations and committed common law fraud in:

   a. intentionally misrepresenting the risks of the toxic effects of the injection of the adenovirus particles;

   b. intentionally failing to inform plaintiff, Paul Gelsinger and plaintiff's decedent regarding the fact that monkeys injected with the virus had become ill and/or died;

   c. intentionally failing to inform Plaintiff, Paul Gelsinger and plaintiff's decedent that patients who had previously participated in the trial suffered serious adverse effects;

   d. intentionally misrepresenting the fact that prior participants in the study had achieved certain efficacy with respect to the treatment of OTC;

   e. intentionally failing to adequately disclose the extent to which Dr. Wilson and the University had a conflict of interest; and

   f. intentionally failing to adequately disclose the financial interest that Dr. Wilson and the University had in relation to the study.

125. The intentional misrepresentations set forth above were done to induce plaintiff's decedent to participate in the gene transfer trial.

126. The misrepresentations set forth above were done with the knowledge that the misrepresentations were false when made.

127. Plaintiff, Paul Gelsinger and plaintiff's decedent, Jesse Gelsinger, justifiably relied upon the misrepresentations set forth above in making the decision as to whether plaintiff's decedent would participate in the gene transfer trial.

128. As a direct and proximate result of defendants' intentional and material misrepresentations as set forth above, plaintiff's decedent, Jesse Gelsinger, participated in the gene transfer trial which ultimately resulted in his death.

129. As a direct and proximate result of the intentional misrepresentations of all defendants named herein, by and through their separate and respective agents, servants, workmen, representatives, physicians, nurses, staff, contractors, medical personnel and employees, said decedent's heirs-at-law and next of kin have in the past been and will in the future continue to be deprived of the earnings, comfort, society and companionship of their said decedent, all to their great loss and detriment.

130. As a direct and proximate result of the foregoing, decedent's wrongful death beneficiaries suffered, are suffering for an indefinite period of time in the future damages, injuries and losses, including but not limited to, a loss of financial support, and the beneficiaries have been wrongfully deprived of the contributions they would have received from decedent, Jesse Gelsinger, including monies which decedent would have provided for such items as clothing, shelter, food, medical care and education.

131. As a direct and proximate result of the foregoing, decedent's wrongful death beneficiaries would have been, continue to be and will be in the future wrongfully deprived of large and various sums of money which decedent would have contributed to their support.

132. As a direct and proximate result of the foregoing, decedent's wrongful death beneficiaries incurred or have been caused to incur and paid large and various expenses various funeral, burial and estate administration.

133. Plaintiff makes claim, on behalf of decedent's heirs-at-law and next-of-kin, for the loss of love, affection, services, earnings, support and all other damages recoverable under the Wrongful Death Statute of the Commonwealth of Pennsylvania.

134. Plaintiff makes claim, on behalf of his decedent's heirs-at-law and next-of-kin, for all damages recoverable under the Survival Statute of the Commonwealth of Pennsylvania.

WHEREFORE, John Gelsinger, as Administrator and Personal Representative of the Estate of Jesse Gelsinger, and Paul Gelsinger, individually, claim of defendants, and each of them respectively, jointly and severally, compensatory damages in excess of Fifty-thousand Dollars ($50,000.00), delay damages pursuant to Pa. R.C.P. 238, punitive damages, interest and allowable costs of suit.

COUNT VII—PUNITIVE DAMAGES

JOHN GELSINGER, AS ADMINISTRATOR AND PERSONAL REPRESENTATIVE OF THE ESTATE OF JESSE GELSINGER v. THE TRUSTEES OF THE UNIVERSITY OF PENNSYLVANIA, CHILDREN'S HOSPITAL OF PHILADELPHIA, CHILDREN'S NATIONAL MEDICAL CENTER, JAMES WILSON, M.D., GENOVO, INC., STEVEN RAPER, M.D., MARK BATSHAW, M.D., WILLIAM N. *KELLEY, M.D., AND ARTHUR CAPLAN, Ph.D.*

135. Plaintiffs incorporate by reference paragraphs 1 through 134 as if fully set forth at length herein.
136. Defendants' actions as set forth above were intentional, wanton, willful and outrageous. Defendants were grossly negligent, and acted with reckless disregard of and with deliberate, callous and reckless indifference to the rights, interests, welfare and safety of plaintiff's decedent.
137. Defendants' intentional, wanton, willful and outrageous actions consisted of, but are not limited to:
   a. intentionally failing to conform to FDA guidelines;
   b. failing to tell the National Institutes of Health Recombinant DNA Advisory Committee ("the RAC") of a change in the way the virus was to be delivered to patients;
   c. ntentionally and recklessly changing the informed consent form from what had been approved by the FDA by removing information concerning the death or illness of several monkeys during a similar study;
   d. intentionally and recklessly failing to report to the FDA that patients prior to Jesse suffered significant liver toxicity which required that the study be put on hold;
   e. intentionally and recklessly failing to follow the study protocol which mandated that in each cohort at least two women be subject to injection before any male;
   f. intentionally and recklessly admitting plaintiff's decedent in the trial when his blood ammonia level on the day before he received the gene transfer exceeded the limit set out in the FDA protocol;
   g. intentionally and recklessly understating the risks of the toxic effects of the injection of the adenovirus particles;
   h. intentionally and recklessly failing to inform plaintiff's decedent regarding the fact that monkeys injected with the virus had become ill and/or died;
   i. intentionally and recklessly failing to inform plaintiff's decedent that patients who had previously participated in the trial suffered serious adverse effects;
   j. intentionally and recklessly misrepresenting the fact that prior participants in the study had achieved certain efficacy with respect to the treatment of OTC;

k. intentionally and recklessly failing to adequately disclose the extent to which Dr. Wilson and the University had a conflict of interest; and

l. intentionally and recklessly failing to inform plaintiff's decedent of the significant financial interest defendants had in the regard to the outcome of the study.

138. Defendants' wanton, willful and outrageous conduct was the direct result of defendants decision to sacrifice patient safety in exchange for the fame and glory which defendants anticipated obtaining if this study and follow up studies using the adenovirus vector were successful.

139. By reason of the wanton, willful and outrageous conduct of defendants, as aforesaid, plaintiff's decedent, Jesse Gelsinger, was caused to sustain the catastrophic injuries which ultimately resulted in his death as described above.

WHEREFORE, John Gelsinger, as Administrator and Personal Representative of the Estate of Jesse Gelsinger, claim of defendants, and each of them respectively, jointly and severally, punitive damages in excess of Fifty-thousand Dollars ($50,000.00), delay damages pursuant to Pa. R.C.P. 238, interest and allowable costs of suit.

COUNT VIII—FRAUD ON THE FOOD AND DRUG ADMINISTRATION

JOHN GELSINGER, AS ADMINISTRATOR AND PERSONAL REPRESENTATIVE OF THE ESTATE OF JESSE GELSINGER AND PAUL GELSINGER v. THE TRUSTEES OF THE UNIVERSITY OF PENNSYLVANIA, JAMES WILSON, M.D., *GENOVO, INC., STEVEN RAPER, M.D. AND MARK BATSHAW, M.D.*

140. Plaintiffs incorporate by reference paragraphs 1 through 139 as if fully set forth at length herein.

141. Defendants, Mark Batshaw, M.D., Steven Raper, M.D., James Wilson, M.D., IHGT, and Genovo intentionally and falsely made numerous fraudulent misrepresentations to the FDA concerning the protocol of the OTC gene transfer experiment.

142. Defendants, Mark Batshaw, M.D., Steven Raper, M.D., James Wilson, M.D., IHGT, and Genovo, failed to disclose that they allowed vectors to sit and/or be stored on lab shelves for 25 months before being tested on animals, making them less potent than they could have been. The vectors administered to the plaintiff's decedent were only stored for two months. The 25-months storage in turn, may have resulted in underestimation of the vectors' potency in humans. Additionally, the animals who received the vector stored for 25 months would have been given a dose of vector from 52.2% to 65.6% below the dose specified in the FDA protocol.

143. Defendants, Mark Batshaw, M.D., Steven Raper, M.D., James Wilson, M.D., IHGT, and Genovo intended for the FDA to approve the gene transfer study based upon those fraudulent misrepresentations.

144. In reliance on those express fraudulent misrepresentations the FDA granted approval of the OTC gene transfer experiment.

145. Defendants altered the FDA approved consent form, deleting any reference to monkeys which became ill and died as a result of receiving a similar vector prior to the experiment.

146. Defendants represented that they would report any adverse or unexpected events associated with the administration of the gene transfer and/or participation in the study, and fraudulently failed to do so.

147. The FDA was without knowledge of the fraudulent nature of the above representations.

148. Were it not for the fraudulent misrepresentations the FDA would not have approved the study, the study would not have been performed, and the plaintiff's decedent would not have been subjected to the experiment which resulted in his death.

149. As a direct and proximate result of the wrongful conduct as alleged above plaintiff's decedent, Jesse Gelsinger, was caused to sustain the catastrophic injuries which resulted in his death.

WHEREFORE, John Gelsinger, as Administrator and Personal Representative of the Estate of Jesse Gelsinger, claim of defendants, and each of them respectively, jointly and severally, punitive damages in excess of Fifty-thousand Dollars ($50,000.00), delay damages pursuant to Pa. R.C.P. 238, interest and allowable costs of suit.

SHERMAN, SILVERSTEIN, KOHL, ROSE & PODOLSKY

By:_____

ALAN C. MILSTEIN
HARRIS L. POGUST

SALTZ, MONGELUZZI, BARRETT& BENDESKY, P.C.

By:_____

ROBERT J. MONGELUZZI
LARRY BENDESKY
Attorneys for Plaintiffs,
John Gelsinger as Administrator of the Estate
of Jesse Gelsinger, and Paul Gelsinger

Timeline for the Advance of Gene Therapy

5000 BC	In selectively breeding crops, humans show some understanding of inheritance.
400 BC	Aristotle develops the theory of pangenesis to explain how traits are transmitted to reproductive cells via particles called *gemules*.
	The Greek philosopher Socrates suggests that some people are born to lead, some to follow, and others to work.
1806	French chemist Louis Nicolas Vauquelin isolates the amino acid aspargine from asparagus.
1812	William Hyde Wollaston finds that urine has a second amino acid.
1820	French chemist Henri Braconnot discovers two natural amino acids, glycine and cystine.
1856	Arthur de Gobineau writes about and promotes racial superiority in his book *The Inequality of the Races.*
1859	Charles Darwin publishes *Origin of Species* in 1859, and some people begin to apply the principles of natural selection to people as groups, or even to whole races.
1866	Austrian monk Gregor Mendel publishes his work on inheritance in pea plants, thereby marking the birth of modern genetics.
1869	Swiss scientist Friedrich Miescher purifies DNA—which he calls *nuclein*—from white blood cells in pus.
1882	British scientist Sir Francis Galton coins the term *eugenics,* based on the Greek word *eugenes,* meaning "good in birth."

	German biologist Walter Fleming discovers chromosomes and names them on the basis of the Greek prefix meaning "color."
1890	German geneticist Albrecht Kossel points to the role of DNA in heredity; the work of Kossel, Mendel, and Miescher is forgotten for the rest of the nineteenth century.
	Nineteenth-century English eugenicist Herbert Spencer agrees with mathematician Thomas Malthus that overpopulation will make life on earth impossible, and the principle of survival of the fittest will prevail.
1899	German scientist Emil Fischer synthesizes many of the 13 known amino acids and isolates three more.
Late 1890s	Alexander Garrod uses the term *inborn errors of metabolism* to describe the disorders shared by members of a family with alkaptonuria, and establishes a new class of diseases based on inheritance.
1901	British biochemist Frederick Gowland Hopkins finds that the amino acid tryptophan plays an important role in the diet.
1902	Biologists rediscover Mendel's research and notice the connection between chromosomes and Mendel's units of heredity.
1905	Biologist William Bateson creates the term *genetics*. The words *gene* and *genotype* emerge in 1909.
	Sex chromosomes are discovered in butterflies and beetles.
1910	U.S. zoologist and geneticist Thomas Hunt Morgan discovers a sex-linked trait in the fruit fly (Drosophila).
1911–1930	In the United States, 24 states pass laws that restrict the right of the "unfit" to have children—either by requiring sterilization or by restricting who may marry.
1912	American geneticist A. H. Sturtevant constructs the first chromosome map, showing genes for specific traits that could be mapped to their location on the four fruit fly chromosomes.
1925	X-rays induce mutations in genes.
1928	Frederick Griffith discovers that a nonvirulent R-type form of the bacterium *pneumococcus* could be turned into the deadly S-type form.
1933	During the German Third Reich, Nazis rise to power and use arguments based on eugenics to justify their "Final Solution," the extermination of Jews and others considered to be inferior.
1944	U.S. geneticists find that DNA is hereditary material, not protein.

1946	U.S. geneticist Hermann Joseph Muller wins the Nobel Prize for Physics or Medicine for mastering how to change genes by radiation.
1940s	Researchers discover that Tay-Sachs disease is caused by a deadly accumulation of fatty acids in the brain that destroys nerve cells.
1944	Oswald Avery replicates the study of Frederick Griffith that showed how one strain of virus can be changed to another form.
1949	U.S. chemist Linus Pauling determines that sickle cell disease is caused by a defect in one of the genes that codes for hemoglobin.
1951	British researcher Rosalind Franklin captures clear X-ray diffraction images of DNA.
1953	American biochemist James Watson and British biophysicist Francis Crick determine at Cambridge University the now famous double-helix structure of DNA. They are awarded a Nobel Prize in 1962 for their efforts.
1956	Joshua Lederberg and colleagues at Rockefeller University discover that when viruses infect a bacterial cell, bits of DNA from the host chromosome are incorporated into viral cells and become incorporated into the offspring of the new viruses.
1961	Crick and South African Sydney Brenner report that trios of DNA bases—called nucleotides—hold the instruction for amino acids that form proteins. U.S. biologist Marshall Nirenberg announces the discovery of the process for unraveling the code of DNA.
1965	Rollin D. Hotchkiss coins the term *genetic engineering* in a talk.
1966	At a symposium titled "Reflection on Research and the Future of Medicine," Joshua Lederberg and Edward Tatum lay out the fundamental ideas that will evolve into the field of gene therapy.
1970	Johns Hopkins University scientist Hamilton Smith discovers the first restriction enzyme called *Hind*III. Paul Berg and fellow Stanford University researchers isolate DNA from the bacterium *Esherischia coli* and the virus SV40 from a monkey.
1970s	Stanley Cohen and Herbert Boyer find that by cutting plasmids from different sources using EcoR1, the two plasmid pieces will adhere.

1971   American Stanfield Rogers is the first to attempt human gene therapy.

NIH researcher Carl R. Merrill begins testing viruses for their ability to transfer genes to cells.

1972   Ernst Freese calls a meeting at NIH to learn what research is being conducted in the field of gene therapy and to possibly develop some ethical guidelines.

1973   U.S. researcher Herb Boyer of Stanford University uses enzymes to cut DNA and splice it into bacterial plasmids that replicate into many copies of an inserted gene.

1978   Modified bacteria produce the first insulin.

1980   Biomedical scientist Martin Cline attempts the first gene therapy using recombinant DNA.

1983   Researchers map the gene for Huntington's disease.

1984   At a meeting in Alta, Utah, the U.S. Department of Energy suggests sequencing the genome as a way to measure exposure to radiation.

Scientists at the University of Cincinnati clone the adenosine deaminase (ADA) gene.

1986   Biochemist Kary Mullis develops the polymerase chain reaction (PCR), which allows researchers to make many copies of a portion of DNA.

1989   The defective gene for Tay-Sachs is found on chromosome 15.

CFTR, the gene that causes cystic fibrosis, is located on the long arm of chromosome 7.

1990   The Human Genome Project begins.

Gene therapy is used to treat a 4-year-old girl with adenosine deaminase deficiency (ADA).

1995   *Hemophilus influenzae,* the bacterium that causes influenza, becomes the first genome of an organism other than a virus to be sequenced.

Craig Venter announces the formation of a new company— Celera Genomics—that would complete the sequencing of the human genome years ahead of the 2005 deadline.

1999   Jesse Gelsinger, an 18-year-old who suffers from the metabolic disorder ornithine transcarbamylase deficiency, dies while participating in a phase I gene therapy trial at the Institute for Human Gene Therapy, located at the University of Pennsylvania.

2000   Several gene therapy protocols undergo testing.

Celera Genomics and the Human Genome Project announce completion of the draft of the human genome.

2001   Gene therapist Philippe Leboulch and colleagues at Harvard Medical School bioengineer mice to contain a human gene that produces the defective hemoglobin that causes sickle cell disease.

Children are born using germ-line transplants.

2002   Professor of Pharmacology Ryszard Kole use gene repair to treat thalassemia.

2005   Dr. Francesca Santoni de Sio of the San Raffaele Institute for Gene Therapy in Milan, Italy, successfully treats six children with ADA and a complete lack of lymphocytes.

Further Reading

"A Cancer Treatment You Can't Get Here." 2006. *BusinessWeek Online.* February 28, 2006. http://www.businessweek.com/print/magazine/ontent/06_10/b3974104. htm?chan=gl.

Access Excellence. 1990. "Gene Therapy—An Overview." *Biotechnology in Perspective.* Washington, DC, Biotechnology Industry Organization. September 13, 2006. http://www.accessexcellence.org/RC/AB/BA/Gene_Therapy_ Overview.html.

"Advancing Gene Therapy." 2006. *FDA Consumer: The Magazine of the U.S. Food and Drug Administration.* 40: 5, 35.

ALSforums. "New ALS Gene Therapy Could Slow Progress of ALS." December 27, 2006. http://www.alsforums.com/als-mnd-news/research-trials/37.html.

Amati, Marissa, et al. 2003. "EMEA and Gene Therapy Medicinal Products Development in the European Union." *Journal of Biomedical Biotechnology* 2003 (1): 3–8.

American Heart Association. February 11, 2000. "Gene Therapy Reverses Heart Disease in Mice." December 18, 2006. http://www.sciencedaily.com/ releases/2000/02/000211082913.htm.

BBC News. December 7, 2000. "Diabetes Gene Therapy Draws Closer." December 18, 2006. http://news.bbc.co.uk/1/hi/sci/tech/1059925.stm.

BPI Reports. June 2005. *BioProcess International.* 3:6, 10.

Bruce, Donald M. 1996. "Moral and Ethical Issues in Gene Therapy." December 25, 2006. http://www.srtp.org.uk/genthpy1.htm.

Burke, Bob, and Barry Epperson. 2003. *W. French Anderson: Father of Gene Therapy.* Oklahoma City: Oklahoma City Heritage Foundation.

Chung, Emily. 2006. "Genetic Brain Disease Cured in Mice." *The Dana Foundation's Brain in the News.* 13: 7.

Chustecka, Zosta. 2006. "Gene Therapy Success in 2 Melanoma Patients Hailed as Breakthrough." *Medscape Medical News.* September 7, 2006. http://www. medscape.com/viewarticle/544154_print.

Crawford, S. Cromwell. 2003. "Hindu Perspectives on Genetic Enhancements in Humans." Loma Linda University Center for Christian Bioethics Update. 18: 4, 2–8.

Dabbah, Roger. June 2005. "Developing Quality Standards." *BioProcess International.* 3:6, 28.

Discovery Zones: Sickle Cell. 2006. *BioExecutive International.* February, 50.

Drouplic, Boro. 2006. "Gene Therapy and Beyond." *Drug Discovery News.* January 11, 2006.

Dykxhoorn, D. M., et al. 2006. "The Silent Treatment: siRNAs as Small Molecule Drugs." *Gene Therapy* 13, 541–52.

Epstein, Ron. 2001. "Genetic Engineering: A Buddhist Assessment." December 31, 2006. http://online.sfsu.edu/~rone/GEessays/GEBuddhism.html.

Fischer, Alain, and Martina Cavazzano–Calvo. 2006. "Whither Gene Therapy?" *The Scientist.* 20: 2, 36–41.

Foubister, Vida. 2005. "Non-Viral Gene Therapy Lights UP." *Drug Discovery Today.* 10: 17, 1133.

France-Presse, Agence. 2006. "South Korean Scientist Eyes Disease Cures from Cloned Dogs." December 21, 2006. http://www.seedmagazine.com/news/2006/12/south_korean_scientist_eyes_di.php.

France-Presse, Agence. 2006. "South Korean Scientists Plan to Clone Monkeys." December 31, 2006. http://www.seedmagazine.com/news/2006/12/south_korean_scientists_plan_t.php.

Fung, H. C., et al. 2006. "A Genome-wide genotyping in Parkinson's disease and neurologically normal controls; first-stage analysis and public release of data." *Lancet Neurology.* 2006 Nov. 5(11): 911–916.

Garber, Ken. 1999. "High Noon for Gene Therapy." *Signals, the Online Magazine of Biotechnology Inquiry.* December 12, 2006. http://www.signalsmag.com/signalsmag.nsf/0/7798E274F16AEB28882567B5006537D6.

"Gene Expression in NF1, the Study of Disease Severity in Adults with NF1." 2006. December 20, 2006. http://www.genome.gov/1601547.

"Gene Therapy." 2006. November 15, 2006. http://en.wikipedia,org/wiki/Gene_therap.

"Gene Therapy." Health A to Z. September 7, 2006. http://www.healthatoz.com/healthyatoz/Atoz/ency/gene_therapy.jsp.

Gene Therapy Advisory Committee. 2005. December 31, 2006. http://www.advisorybodies.doh.uk/genetics/gtac/.

"Gene Therapy Inhibits Epilepsy." November 15, 2006. http://media.prnewswire.com/en/jps?searchtype=full&option=headline&criter.

"Gene Therapy Regenerates Functioning Auditory Hair Cells." 2005. April 6, 2006. www.med.umich.edu/opm/newspage/2005/haircell.htm.

"Gene Therapy Used to Correct Myeloid Immunodeficiency." 2006. November 7, 2006. http://www.medscape.com/viewarticle/528994_print.

"Gene Therapy Works in Mice to Prevent Blindness that Strikes Boys." August 2, 2005 news release, University of Florida Office of News and Communications.

Goyenvalle, A., et al. 2005. "Highly efficient exon-skipping and sustained correction for muscular dystrophy using an adeno-associated viral vector." Program and abstracts of the American Society of Gene Therapy Annual Meeting; June 1–5, 2005; St. Louis, Missouri.

Guidotti, J. E., et al. 1999. "Adenoviral Gene Therapy of the Tay-Sachs Disease in Hexosaminidase A-deficient Knockout Mice." *Human Molecular Genetics* 8, 5: 831–38.

Harris, Louis and Associates. 1992. March of Dimes Survey of Attitudes of American Adults toward Using Gene Therapy. Poll conducted in spring 1992.

Harris, Michael. 2006. "Book Review: Michael Crichton's *Next.*" December 27, 2006. http://www.calendarlive.com/books/reviews/cl-et-book28nov28,0, 373911,print.story?coll.

Holmes, Bob. 2003. "Gene Therapy May Switch Off Huntington's" *New Scientist. com.* 10: 32 March. November 24, 2006. http://www.newscientist.com/ article.ns?id=dn3493&print=true.

Human Gene Therapy—A Background Paper. 1984. Washington, DC: U.S. Congress. Office of Technology Assessment. OTA-BP-BA-32 December.

Huntley, Ola M. Transcript of a presentation at *Public Forum on Gene Therapy* sponsored by the National Institute on Child Health and Human Development, Masur Auditorium, National Institutes of Health, Bethesda, MD, November 21, 1983, pp. 158–69.

IslamOnline.net. December 25, 2006. http://www.islamonline.net/servlet/Satellite? pagename=IslamOnline-English-Ask_Schola.

Johns Hopkins Institutions Alumni and Friends. 2005. "Gene Therapy Alternative to Calcium Channel Blockers for Heart Disease Works in Animals." December 18, 2006. https://hopkinsnet.jhu.edu/servlet/page?_pageid=935&_dad= portal30p&_schema=PORT.

Journal of Gene Medicine. 2006. December 31, 2006. http://abedia.com/wiley/ countries.php.

Kelly, Evelyn B. 2007. *Stem Cells.* Westport, CT: Greenwood Press.

Kelly, Evelyn B. 2006. *Obesity.* Westport, CT: Greenwood Press.

Kevles, D. J. 1984. "Annals of Eugenics: A Secular Faith." Series of four articles published in *The New Yorker.* October 8, pp. 51ff; Oct. 15, pp. 52ff; Oct. 22, pp. 92ff; Oct 29, pp. 51ff.

Khamsi, Roxanne. May 2006. "Diabetes Gene Therapy Carried by Bubbles in the Blood." NewScientist.com. December 18, 2006. http://www.newscientist. com/article.ns?id=dn9174&print=true.

Learn.Genetics. 2006. November 15, 2006. http://learn.genetics.utah.edu/units/ genetherapy/gttargets.

"Learning about Retinitis Pigmentosa." December 20, 2006. http://www.genome. gov/pfv.cfm?pageID=13514348.

Levasseur, Dana. et al. 2003. "Correction of Sickle Cell Disease: Lentiviral/ antisickling β-globin Gene Transduction of Unmobilized, Purified Hematopoietic Stem Cells." *Blood.* 102: 4312–9.

Lewis, Ricki. 1997. *Human Genetics: Concepts and Applications.* Dubuque, IA: Wm. C. Brown.

Lyon, Jeff. 1996. *Altered Fates: Gene Therapy and the Retooling of Human Life.* New York: W.W. Norton.

Maloney, Michael, et al. 2006. "Safety and Efficacy of Ultraviolet-A Light-activated Gene Transduction for Gene Therapy of Articular Cartilage Defects." *Journal of Bone and Joint Surgery.* 88: 753–61.

Martino S., et al. 2005. "A Direct Gene Transfer Strategy via Brain Internal Capsule Reverses the Biochemical Defect of Tay-Sachs Disease." *Human Molecular Genetics* 14 (15): 2113–23.

McElheny, Victor. 2006. "The Human Genome Project." *The Scientist* 20: 2, 42–8.

McKusick, V. A. 1984. *Mendelian Inheritance in Man.* 6th ed. Baltimore: Johns Hopkins Press.

"Oxford Biomedica Presents Encouraging Data for Parkinson's Treatment." 2006. December 29, 2006. http://drugresearcher.com/news/ng.asp?id=72046-oxford-biomedica-parkinson-s-pr.

Pai, S. I., et al. 2005. Prospects of RNA Interference Therapy for Cancer. *Gene Therapy* 13: 464–77.

Pawliuk, R., and P. Leboulch. 2001. "Correction of Sickle Cell Disease in Transgenic Mouse Models by Gene Therapy. *Science* 294 (Dec. 14): 2368–71.

Penman, Danny. 2002. "Subtle Gene Therapy Tackles Blood Disorder." *New Scientist* 16: 26, 11.

Reader Roundtable. January 2006. From e-letter of *BioProcess International.* January 20, 2006. BPI_Editors@xmr3.com.

Reaney, Patricia. 2006. "New Human Gene Map Shows Surprising Difference." November 24, 2006. http://articles.news.aol.com/news/_a/new-human-gene-map-shows-surprising/200611221.

Rosner, Fred. 2006. "Judaism, Genetic Screening, and Genetic Therapy." December 31, 2006. http://www.jewishvirtuallibrary.org/jsource/Judaism/genetic.html.

Rush University Medical Center. 2005. "Rush Physicians Using Gene Therapy for Heart Patients with Moderate to Severe Chest Pains Who Do Not Benefit from Other Treatments." December 18, 2006. http://www.sciencedaily.com/releases/2005/02/05020505115737.htm.

"Sangamo Biosciences Creates Genetically Modified Immune Cells that Resist HIV Infections in Lab Test." 2005. January 4, 2007. http://www.thebody.com/kaiser/2005/dec20_05.hiv_resistant_cells.html.

Santoni de Sio, F., and L. Nandini. 2005. "Lentiviral gene transfer into hSC is enhanced by early-acting cytosines without impairing stem cell properties and involves cellular responses distinct from cell cycle control." Program and abstracts of the American Society of Gene Therapy Annual Meeting; June 1–5, 2005; St. Louis, Missouri.

Schlager, Neil, ed. 2000. *Science and Its Times: Understanding the Social Significance of Scientific Discovery,* vol. 7, 1900–2000. Detroit: Gale Group.

SRIS Science and Religion Information Service. 2001. "Gene Therapy and Sickle Cell Disease: Religious Perspectives." December 25, 2006. http://www.sris.info/brief.ep.html?id=15.

Sweeney, Rory. 2005. "Sending Genes to Save a Child." *The Dana Foundation's Brain in the News.* September, vol. 12, 9, 1–2.

Tanner, Lindsey. December 22, 2006. "Desiging Babies with Defects Unethical?" Ocala, FL, *Ocala Star-Banner*, vol. 64, no. 113, Section 1A, pp. 1, 4. Associated Press story written in Chicago.

"Targeting a Key Enzyme with Gene Therapy Reversed Course of Alzheimer's Disease in Mouse Models." Press release from Salk Institute. December 16, 2006. http://www.eurekalert.org/pub_releases/2005-09/si-tak092005.php.

Thobaben, Robert, et al. 2006. *Issues in American Political Life: Money, Violence, and Biology.* Upper Saddle River, NJ: Pearson/Prentice Hall.

Thompson, Larry. 1994. *Correcting the Code.* New York: Simon and Schuster.

Tuszynski, M. H., et al. 2005. "A Phase I Clinical Trial of Nerve Growth Factor Gene Therapy for Alzheimer's Disease." *Nature Medicine.*

UK Department of Health. 2005. "UK Leads Europe in Gene Therapy Trials." December 31, 2006. http://www.dh.gov.uk/PublictionsAndStatistics/PressReleases/PressReleasesNotices/fs/e.

University of Florida News. 2006. "UF Scientists Test Improved Gene Therapy Method for Hereditary Heart Conditions." December 18, 2006. http://news.ufl.edu/2006/07/27/heart-gene-2/.

"VIRxSYS Completes HIV Gene Therapy Study." 2005. January 4, 2007. http://drugresearcher.com/news/ng.asp?id=59798-virsys-completes-hiv.

Vogelstein, B., and K. W. Kinzler. 2004. "Cancer Genes and the Pathways They Control." *Nature Medicine* 10: 789–99.

World Council of Churches. 1984. *Manipulating Life: Ethical Issues in Genetic Engineering.* Geneva: Church and Society World Council of Churches.

Young, Emma. 2002. "Miracle gene therapy trial halted." New Scientist.com News Service 14: 30. November 24, 2006. http://www.newscientist.com/article.ns?id=dn2878&print=true.

Web Sites

FDA: http://www.fda.gov/cber/

NIH: http://www.nih.gov

Council for Responsible Genetics: www.gene-watch.org

Campaign for Responsible Transplantation: http://www.crt-online.org

Protect your medical rights: http://www.dialogmedical.com/ic.htm

Clinical trials guide: http://www.jsonline.com/alive/ap/apr02/ap-medical-experim 041502.asp

Database on clinical trials: http://www.clinicaltrials.gov

Public information on gene therapy from the National Cancer Institute: http://cis.
    nci.nih.gov/fact/7_18.htm
An overview of the history of gene therapy: http://www.ornl.gov/TechResources/
    Human_Genome/medicine/genetherapy.html
Concise articles simply written: http://www.accessexcellence.org/RC/AB/BA/
    Gene_Therapy_Overview.html

Glossary

adeno-associated viruses (AAVs) Small, single-stranded DNA viruses that can insert their genetic material at a specific site

adenoviruses (ADs) A class of viruses with double-stranded DNA genomes that cause respiratory, intestinal, and eye infections in humans. They can efficiently enter most cells and infect stationary cells.

Alzheimer's disease (AD) A progressive brain disease marked by dementia and loss of memory. The brain of a person with Alzheimer's disease is characterized by plaque and neurofibrillary tangles.

amino acid An organic compound containing an NH_2 amino and a COOH carboxyl group

antisense gene therapy A type of gene therapy that turns off a mutated gene in a cell by targeting the mRNA transcripts copied from the gene

autologous transplant A transplant in which a patient's own cells are removed, genetically corrected, and then placed back into the body

autosomes Also called **somatic** or body chromosomes

bacteriophage A simple piece of DNA that attaches to a bacterium and injects its own DNA into the cell

capsid A small vesicle that connects with cell receptors and is drawn into the cell

catalyze The speeding up of the rate of a chemical reaction

CFTR gene Cystic fibrosis transmembrane conductance regulator, the gene associated with cystic fibrosis

chromosome From the Greek root words *chromo,* meaning "color," and *soma,* meaning "body." In humans, 23 pairs carry genes, the elements of heredity.

cloning The process of making multiple copies of a single gene in the laboratory

codon The three-base sequence that codes for an amino acid

cystic fibrosis An autosomal recessive disorder in which the glands do not function and mucus builds up in the lungs

cytosine The signaling molecule produced by T lymphocytes that coordinates an organism's immune response

deoxyribonucleic acid (DNA) The double-stranded molecule containing hereditary information in almost all organisms

endocytosis The process whereby sugar and some hormone molecules have receptors that gain entry to the cell

enzyme A protein that acts to facilitate the building up or tearing down of biochemical reactions

eugenics The practice of attempting to improve the human race by selective breeding

exon The region in a gene that encodes protein

expressivity The extent to which a person has the signs or symptoms of a genetic disease

ex vivo (or in vitro) gene therapy Cells are modified outside the body and then transplanted back into the body

gene The portion of the DNA molecule that acts like the hard drive of a computer and stores information in discrete chunks of genetic information.

gene gun A device that shoots DNA-coated gold particles into a cell using high-pressure gas

genetic marker A particular gene or DNA base sequence associated with a particular chromosome

genome The entire complement of genes in an organism's DNA

gene therapy A set of approaches designed to correct the defective genes responsible for disease development

germ-line cells The reproductive cells, such as sperm or ova

hemoglobin The protein that carries oxygen in red blood cells and gives the cells their red color

Huntington's disease An inherited neurological condition caused by a single gene defect

intron A section of a gene that is noncoding

in vivo gene therapy Genes are changed in cells still in the body

lentiviruses A special group of viruses, of which HIV is a member

liposome A round lipid body whose shell may be filled to deliver substances to a particular organ

messenger RNA (mRNA) A gene template used by ribosomes and other components of translation to synthesize a protein

monogenic Involving only a single gene

nucleus The central part of the cell where cells activities are regulated

nucleotide A polymer containing one or more phosphate groups linked to the 5´-sugar of the ribose sugar, of which DNA and RNA are examples

oligonucleotide A short, single-stranded piece of DNA

ornithine transcarbamylase (OTC) deficiency An X-linked defect associated with a specific enzyme deficiency in the nitrogen cycle in which ammonia builds up, causing mental deterioration and liver failure

pangenesis Aristotle's explanation that traits are passed to the mother through particles called "gemules"

Parkinson's disease A neurological disease characterized by loss of dopamine in the striatum of the brain. The disease causes tremors and other neurological problems.

penetrance The expression of a gene in a population in which some organisms are affected and others that carry the gene are not affected

phagocyte A white blood cell, important to the immune system, that engulfs foreign cells, viruses, and debris

plasmid A small, circular piece of DNA bacteria that is separate from the normal chromosomal DNA of the bacterium

point mutation A change in only one nucleotide

polygenic Involving many genes

polymerase chain reaction (PCR) A chain reaction in which copies of DNA are mechanically made

polymorphic Having two or more distinct forms that exist within a single breeding population of a species

primer An engineered piece of DNA comprising about 18 to 24 bases and made to lie between a different stretch of DNA that is destined to be copied

promoter A sequence of DNA to which RNA binds to promote transcription

protein Substance made of linking amino acids

proteome Complete set of the proteins that make up an organism

restriction enzyme An enzyme that has the ability to recognize a specific nucleotide sequence and cut or cleave the nucleic acid at that point

retrovirus A virus that converts its DNA to RNA once it is in the cell

reverse transcriptase An enzyme that synthesizes RNA into DNA (the reverse of the usual flow of DNA into RNA)

ribonucleic acid (RNA) A polynucleotide in which uracil replaces cytosine in the template of the bases

ribozyme RNA molecule that behaves like an enzyme, acting like scissors to cut RNA

RNA interference Involves a natural defense mechanism against viruses. In this process, short pieces of double-stranded RNA—called *short interfering RNAs (siRNAs)*—trigger the degrading of other RNA in the cell with a matching sequence.

sickle cell anemia/sickle cell disease (SCD) A condition in which a single molecule of valine has replaced the glutamic acid molecule in one of the chains of the hemoglobin molecule, the protein that carries oxygen in red blood cells

somatic chromosome Also called "body chromosome"

splice site The area where the cell cuts and pastes the RNA.

stem cells Cells found in embryos and various body parts that can differentiate into a wide variety of cell types

stop codon A series of triplets that indicates the ending of a gene

T lymphocytes Cells of the immune system

transcription Process in which a complementary messenger RNA (mRNA) molecule is formed from a single-stranded DNA template

translation Process in which the nucleotide sequence of an mRNA molecule is used as a template to direct the synthesis of a protein

vector A virus or plasmid that delivers therapeutic material into cells

virsome Substance that combines a liposome with an inactivated HIV or influenza virus

INDEX

ABOUT THE AUTHOR

EVELYN B. KELLY is a writer specializing in health and environmental topics. She is a co-author of *The Skeletal System* volume in the Greenwood Human Body Systems series and the author of the *Stem Cells* volume in the Health and Medical Issues Today series.